Robert Graves

The Golden Years of Irish Medicine

Selwyn Taylor

Editor-in-Chief: Hugh L'Etang

Royal Society of Medicine Services Limited

Royal Society of Medicine Services Limited
1 Wimpole Street London W1M 8AE
7 East 60th Street New York NY 10022

British Library Cataloguing in Publication Data

Taylor, S.
   Robert Graves
   1. Medicine. Graves, Robert 1796–1853
   I. Title II. Series
   610' .92,4
   ISBN 0-905958-90-X

Editorial and production services by Diane Crofter-Harris, Devizes, Wiltshire

Design and typesetting by Mehmet Hussein/Medilink Design

Printed in Great Britain by Henry Ling Ltd, at the Dorset Press, Dorchester

Contents

Illustrations

Foreword

This is the story of an Irish physician whose name is still a household word among doctors; he is rightly remembered, but for the wrong reasons. The complaint to which his name is applied by English speaking doctors, Graves' disease, was first described ten years earlier by another physician, Caleb Hillier Parry of Bath. Despite all this it is very proper to remember Robert James Graves for he was a brilliant doctor who revolutionised the medical practice of his day and introduced a method of teaching students at the bedside which still continues to be the mainstay of medical education.

Graves was an outstanding scholar all his life and whatever subject he touched, biology, anatomy, chemistry and epidemiology, not to mention clinical medicine, he added distinction to it. He had a flair for foreign languages and was fluent in French, German and Italian. He was exceedingly well read and was a great traveller in Europe, always anxious to keep abreast of developments in other countries.

The period in which he lived, the first half of the nineteenth century, was one of great biological awareness and he brought a keen critical mind to the advances then being made. He practised in Dublin when that city was the medical Mecca of the world and during a period when such distinguished men as Cheyne, Stokes, Corrigan, Colles, Adams and Wilde were his colleagues and immediate contemporaries. Little wonder that those times are still referred to as the golden years of Irish medicine.

My old mentor and friend, the Boston physician Howard Means, started to write this book in the 1960s, but was unable to get very far by the time he died. I rashly undertook to complete it, but it has taken far longer than I ever dreamt, some twenty five years in all. One of the prime difficulties was that Graves was a very private person and few of his letters and personal things have survived. However, he was a prolific author of medical works and through these and the comments of his friends and contemporaries it has been possible to piece together the portrait of a fascinating character.

Selwyn Taylor

Trippets
Bosham
West Sussex   1988

Acknowledgements

This book has been so long in gestation that it would be impossible to mention everyone by name who has helped in providing information over the years, but I do acknowledge most gratefully all the assistance I have received. There are some, however, whom I would like to mention because they have given outstanding help.

First and foremost Carol Means for supplying all the relevant papers of the late Howard Means who started the project, and for her constant warm friendship; the Librarians of the Royal College of Surgeons of England, in particular Eustace Cornelius and his successor Ian Lyle; the Royal College of Physicians of Ireland; the Royal College of Surgeons in Ireland; The Royal College of Physicians of London; the National Library of Ireland; and Trinity College Library, Dublin.

Professor Niall O'Higgins of St Vincent's Hospital, Dublin, has been enormously helpful in many ways providing information, assistance and unfailing hospitality. Mr J McAuliffe Curtin when President of the Royal College of Surgeons in Ireland was of particular help, Professor Havsner of the Rigshospitalet, Copenhagen, provided Johannes Colsmann's particulars and Mr Victor Lane, President of the RCSI in 1984 produced invaluable material about the Meath Hospital of which he was senior surgeon, as was his father before him.

The Most Revd George Sims, now of Dublin, and Dean Maurice Talbot of Banagher unravelled a number of problems about the Graves family and their homes. Baron Robertson of Strathloch, of Clonegal Castle (the Revd Lawrence Durdin-Robertson) provided much of the early history of the Irish branch of the Graves family and his hospitality went so far on one occasion as to invite us to search in the castle's attics. Mrs Binney of Kiftsgate House, Mickleton and doctors Donald and Jennifer Olliff of Chipping Camden provided information about those original Graves and their home in Mickleton, Gloucestershire from whom the Irish branch of the family descended.

Dr John Hayes, Director of the National Portrait Gallery assisted with the search concerning the story of Graves and Turner and Rosaleen Ellis delved deeply into the Turner records at the Clore Gallery extension at the Tate Gallery. Robin Price of the Wellcome Foundation for the History of Medicine provided material on Stokes and Graves. The Royal Society gave the list of sponsors and their nomination for Graves' election as FRS.

My friend, fellow student and old shipmate, John Naish, read the earlier drafts and offered helpful criticism just when it was needed. Finally, over and above all else it is my wife who has aided and abetted me at every stage of the endeavour and it is to her, out of thanks for this unstinting assistance, that I dedicate the finished work.

Selwyn Taylor.

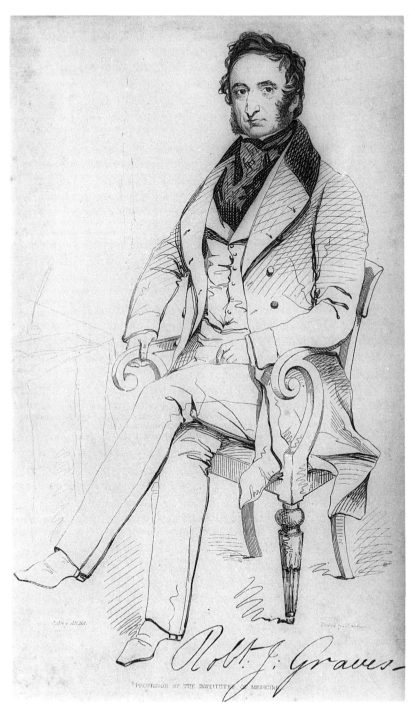

Portrait of Robert Graves by Charles Grey RHA. By Courtesy of the National Gallery of Ireland.

Robert James Graves MD FRS
1796–1853

1796	Born on March 28 at Holles Street, Dublin to the Revd Richard and Eliza Graves.
1815	BA Trinity College Dublin.
1818	Graduates MB at Trinity.
1818-1820	Studies abroad in London, Göttingen, Berlin, Copenhagen and Edinburgh. Visits Italy.
1820	Licentiate, Royal College of Physicians of Ireland.
1821	Appointed Physician to the Meath Hospital, Dublin. Marries Matilda Jane Eustace.
1823	Elected Fellow of the Royal College of Physicians of Ireland. Leads team of doctors to treat typhus epidemic in Galway.
1824	Co-founder of the Park Street School of Medicine. Appointed Lecturer in Institutes of Medicine and Toxicology.
1825	Wife Matilda Jane and young daughter Eliza Drewe both die.
1826	Marries Sarah Jane Brinkley daughter of John Brinkley, Professor of Astronomy at Trinity and Astronomer Royal in Ireland, who in the same year becomes Bishop of Cloyne.
1827	Elected King's Professor in Institutes of Medicine. The first full-time Chair of Medicine in Ireland. Wife Sarah Jane dies and their child Sara-Jane.
1830	Third marriage; to Anna Grogan daughter of the Revd William Grogan of Slaney Park, Baltinglass, Co. Wicklow. She is to outlive him for twenty years, dying in 1873.
1835	Describes three cases of toxic goitre at a lecture at the Meath Hospital, published in the London Medical and Surgical Journal, 7 (part 2), pp 516-7. Treats 300 cases of typhus and typhoid at the Meath.
1841	Resigns from his Chair of Medicine
1843-1844	President of the Royal College of Physicians of Ireland. Resigns from staff of the Meath hospital.
1849	Elected Fellow of the Royal Society.
1853	Dies of liver cancer at home in Dublin on March 20.

For Ruth

Chapter 1

Introduction

The sea mist seeped into St Stephen's Green as it drifted in from Dublin Bay and as soon as we drove out of the garage, although it was nine o'clock in the morning, it was essential to turn on the headlights of the car, not only to identify ourselves to the other traffic, but also so as to try and read the road signs for this was to be a voyage of exploration. Ruth my wife was, as always, the navigator and an expert into the bargain, but we had only been able to find a map with a scale of twelve miles to the inch which, with the fog, added to our difficulties. We headed due west, hoping to discover Cloghan Castle near the little town of Banagher on the banks of the river Shannon.

As soon as we left the city limits the traffic dwindled to a mere trickle but then Irish roads are so often deserted. All too soon, in the murk, the verges closed in on us until it was a single track with occasional wider passing places. Some way behind us I could see in the driving mirror the loom of a truck's headlamps and no matter what my speed the other driver kept following at a steady distance. It was a little uncanny, insulated as we were from the outside world by dense mist, never seeing any other vehicle except for the hazy headlamps of the big lorry pounding along in the distance behind us. So we progressed, not identifying any landmark on the map for some twenty miles and then, discretion being the better part of valour, we pulled into the verge on one of the passing places to try and work out, by means of dead reckoning on the map, where on earth we had landed ourselves. The truck thundered past and then immediately his brake lights appeared in the mist and he stopped, the cab door opened and down got the driver, a big man who strode back to where we sat and thrusting his head in the window said, in a rich Irish brogue, "You'll be lost now".

We certainly were! But where else in the whole of Europe can you expect to find such courtesy and thoughtfulness. Why were we looking for Cloghan Castle? The Irish, we soon discovered, are always curious. We explained that we were looking for the one time home of Robert Graves the famous Dublin doctor. No, he had never heard of Cloghan Castle, but yes he knew Banagher well. Indeed, he was heading that way now and if we would follow him he would show us the main street of the town where we should ask the way to the castle. We thanked him and not long after he was waving goodbye to us from his cab window as we drew in and parked the car at the entrance to the local hotel for an overdue Guinness and ploughman's lunch of bread and cheese. Not, however, before noting, as we walked down the high street, a signpost pointing towards Cloghan Castle.

This all leads to the question: why should a retired London surgeon and his doctor wife be trying to follow in the footsteps of an Irish physician who lived 150 years ago—the famous Robert James Graves who initiated the Golden Years of Irish Medicine as they have come to be known and after whom the disease is named which is today recognised as due to overactivity of the thyroid gland which sits so accessibly in the front of the neck. The eponym Graves' disease is used by doctors the world over and none appears ever to have tackled the problem of writing his biography.

The answer to this question arose in the years 1948–1949 when I enjoyed a year's sabbatical leave, thanks to a Rockefeller travelling fellowship, to work at Harvard Medical School and the Massachusetts General Hospital in Boston where there is a world famous thyroid clinic, at that time under the direction of the chief of medicine, Doctor Howard Means. I had been fascinated by the thyroid, that little H-shaped endocrine gland in the neck which secretes its hormones into the blood stream, since reading physiology at Oxford in the early 1930s and later at King's College Hospital in London. In the 1939–1945 war I served as a surgeon in the Royal Navy where there was little scope for such things, but when I found myself once more a civilian I returned to my first love of academic surgery and, joining the staff of Hammersmith Hospital in London, it was again possible to continue a research programme in the medical school, later to be renamed the Royal Postgraduate Medical School.

There was no better place for me to go in 1948 than the MGH as it is always known, both for its excellent research laboratory facilities and the stimulus of working with such colleagues. In addition there was the richness of the clinical material available due to the patients who came not only from Boston and the rest of the USA but also from all over the world, attracted to its Thyroid Clinic which blossomed under the direction of Howard Means. That I, Ruth, and our three-year-old son should be able to study abroad in those early post-war years was entirely due to the award of the Rockefeller Fellowship and this in turn was thanks to Ian Aird, the Professor of Surgery in the Postgraduate Medical School. He was the kindest, most generous of men and a brilliant teacher of surgery who did everything possible to aid his young assistants to pursue their own investigations. How tragic that his remarkable talents and exuberant happy extroversion should in the end lead him to take his own life in a sudden fit of depression in 1957.

I think that in retrospect it is fair to say that for any young surgeon of 35 with wife and three-year-old son in lodgings in a foreign city this was, in addition to being a time of intellectual stimulus, also one of considerable insecurity. Howard Means, a warm hearted, sparkling and witty New Englander must have sensed this, for he became not only mentor but friend and his home an oasis where there was always a warm welcome. Later he made a trip to London to attend the International Goitre Conference and for good measure went on afterwards to Ireland to see the land from which his forbears originally emigrated to the USA.

He certainly saw it through rose tinted spectacles, being driven round the country by a charming young Irish medical student. His trip was completed by a visit to Trinity College Dublin and of course the Meath Hospital, where Graves first saw patients suffering from what was later to be designated Graves' disease. The Royal College of Physicians was proud to open all its doors to Dr Means and, as a special treat, included a visit to Mount Jerome cemetery where due homage was paid at Graves' tomb. Fortunately one of the Fellows carried out a preliminary reconnaissance on the previous day only to find the head stone completely overgrown and undecipherable, but this was soon remedied before the official party arrived. Dr Means has recorded this visit to the land of his forefathers in a charming article 'A Sentimental Journey' in the news sheet of the Massachusetts General Hospital in January 1961 and it was there and then that he decided to spend some of his time in retirement writing the life of his hero Graves.

When he returned home, Howard Means set to work on what he hoped would be a definitive biography; he was an experienced author whose numerous works revealed skill and charm, his monograph on *The Thyroid* having become the standard text on the subject, worldwide. He wrote to his Irish friends for suitable bibliography and consulted all he could find in the medical library in Boston, usually an unfailing source of material, but all he could find was the bare bones of a man, he needed to clothe them with flesh and blood. He never succeeded in finding anything personal; letters and the like had all been destroyed, and this seemed to be the main reason why nothing previously had been published. He settled down to read through Graves' magnum opus, *Clinical Medicine*. I have the two volumes in front of me, heavily annotated by him; there are over 1300 pages in the two volumes, and some of his remarks are very shrewd and often amusing. He became particularly interested in the story of the great potato famine of the 1840s and then, in the 1960s he returned to Dublin where I met him quite by chance in Sir Patrick Dun's Hospital for I was at that time external examiner in surgery for University College Dublin. On that occasion he came on to London and it was like old times entertaining him in our home.

My final encounter with Howard Means was when he lay dying

in the MGH in Boston; he had had little further success with writing
Graves' life. Would I finish it for him? Of course I would. But I little
realised then what a near impossible task I had set myself at that
time. It is sadly true that, just as Howard had already discovered,
so much of what a biographer needs to consult was missing, and now
fully twenty years have elapsed before the task which I so readily
promised to perform has been completed. The search has led my
wife and me into strange places and even stranger encounters with
fascinating people.

There are many reasons why it has taken so long to write this life
of Graves. Primarily, it was to be many years before I retired from
active surgical practice. Meanwhile, the medical school was rebuilt
and then I accepted the deanship which meant a huge additional
load of administrative duties, on top of which there was a steady
flow of young surgeons coming, often from overseas, to work with
me. However the best answer to the question of why anyone should
want to reconstruct the life story of Graves in the first place is very
properly given in Howard Means' own account of his 'Sentimental
Journey' to Ireland in 1960. The title 'Sentimental Journey' is of
course borrowed from Sterne who was born in Clonmel, County
Tipperary to an Irish mother.

This is how Means puts it:

"The name of Robert Graves", he says "is known to every English
speaking member of our profession, and to many others. The
American Goiter Society has emblazoned his countenance upon its
letterhead, but why? There can be no doubt that it is chiefly, if not
entirely, for his classical and excellent description of exophthalmic
goiter that he is known. Graves, however, was not the first to
recognise this syndrome. His first published report on it was in
1835, but Caleb Hillier Parry of Bath had preceded this by twenty
years, and Guiseppe Flajani had reported cases of goiter and violent
heart action as early as 1802. All these physicians, together with the
German, von Basedow, who described the malady in 1840, and with
one or two others, have served eponymic roles with respect to
exophthalmic goiter. If one wanted to be utterly fair-minded,
eponymically, perhaps one should call it Flajani-Parry-Graves-
Basedow disease. This isn't much worse than Hand-Schüller-Chris-
tian disease, or Charcot-Marie-Tooth type of progressive muscular
atrophy. But why an eponym at all? Simply because the purpose of
a term is to convey meaning, and in this case by long association the
eponyms have come to convey, more concisely and clearly than any
descriptive appellation can do, the concept of a disease entity. Long
usage decrees, moreover, that in English it shall be 'Graves' and in
continental languages, 'Basedow's' disease, nor must we forget that
before any of these worthies, artists had observed the prominent
eyes and enlarged necks, for they have left records of them in paint."

Means continues "The chief point to make now, however, is that

Graves, had he never touched upon exophthalmic goiter, still would be one of medicine's famous figures. As a clinical teacher he was outstanding. His published volumes of lectures on clinical medicine constitute a medical text of first rank. Being lectures, they are somewhat chattier than modern textbooks of medicine, but they are systematic and comprehensive, nevertheless. Graves was evidently a physician of very wide clinical experience, but with a profound interest in the underlying sciences upon which he drew freely for explanations of clinical phenomena. Thus, in his studies on inflammation he had constantly in mind the physiological events taking place in the capillary and arteriolar vessels. He always made every effort to consider the true nature of morbid change in designing treatment to correct it, and he was not one to accept prevailing theories uncritically. Often he dissented, and gave logical reasons for doing so."

Finally Means comes to what I believe to be Graves' most important contribution, his methods of clinical teaching. The old days of walking the wards so beloved of the Victorian novelist were at last numbered and Graves, unlike his colleagues, did not strike a god-like pose when teaching at the bedside. In those days the consultant, with his jealously guarded honorary position on the staff of what was always, in everything but name, a charitable or poor-law institution, passed from bedside to bedside holding forth on the various patterns of disease as evidenced in 'his' patients. He prescribed empirical remedies; he did not expect to be asked questions nor, least of all, have his dogma questioned. Enter Graves, and he carefully appointed his own clerks and treated them like junior colleagues, discussing diagnosis at the bedside, and there is no doubt that he was a wonderfully good and astute diagnostician. He expected treatment to have been already prescribed, for which he always wanted to know the rationale. In Graves' own words "You come here to convert theoretical into practical knowledge" and Means comments, "He was indoctrinating his students in these matters and this, he implied, could not be done sitting on benches listening to lectures, but only at the bedside, and, what is more, in a responsible role at the bedside. So he invented the clinical clerkship, and put it to use in the Meath Hospital in the early 1820s. He did not actually claim to have invented it, and said he got the idea from Germany. Nevertheless, if this is so, he at least improved upon it. In any event, there was nothing of the sort elsewhere in the UK at that time, nor for many years after he had it in successful operation in Dublin. Without such a system as the clinical clerkship, Graves maintained, a man becomes a practitioner of medicine without ever having learned to practise. He has had no 'experience', because he has at no time been charged with the responsibility of investigating a case for himself and by himself, because at no time has he been called on to make a diagnosis unassisted by others, and above all, because he has never been obliged to act upon that diagnosis, and prescribed the method of treatment". Howard Means concludes his comments on Graves' innovation in the teaching of doctors with the pithy statement, "Here is something to which modern medical educators can appropriately pay homage".

Thus it was that we set off to explore this remarkable man who lived from 1796 to 1853 by researching his background and that of his colleagues and contemporaries. We sought out the surroundings in which he grew up and in which his talents blossomed. He was a prolific writer but what has been handed down to us is almost exclusively that which was published and that means it concerned such subjects as the diagnosis and treatment of disease, natural science of almost every complexion, education and philosophy; but when it comes to personal matters such as letters, hardly more than a handful have survived. He was by any standards a very private individual. His descendants have told us that the family are known to have destroyed one collection of personal correspondence because they believed it reflected badly on their image.

However we have had nothing but help and courtesy from those descendants we have been able to trace and we always long for, hope and even expect that one day we shall uncover a cache of letters which will shed more light on this fascinating man. The son is father of the man and we have traced the people from whom he sprang and studied their lives. Many of them were very distinguished in their own right. A study of his teachers tells us much about their pupil and in turn when reading through the amazing amount of printed material which Graves himself has left us, it is sometimes possible to find out as much about the author as about the subject on which he wrote. I have attempted to seek out everything Graves produced and read it, so that much that is written here has a medical context if not a medical content, but for those who ask the question: was the book written for doctors and those who work in medicine? the answer is not *only* for them. So many readers today have a good working knowledge of scientific matters, and little if any specialised knowledge is necessary to understand what has been written here.

The first half of the nineteenth century in Dublin has earned itself the title of the Golden Years of Irish Medicine and when one makes a roll-call of the doctors and surgeons who shone at that time (Cheyne, Stokes, Adams, Corrigan, Colles and Wilde, to mention only some of the brightest stars of the day), it is surprising how many of their names are still household words wherever medicine is practised. Graves stands out like a giant among them and they acknowledged him as such. Here then is the story of a brilliant doctor, scholar, scientist, polymath and author who was an outstanding teacher.

Chapter 2

Graves' Forbears

Often when engaged in research one sets off on a likely line of investigation only to make some different but happy discovery quite by accident. Serendipidity, Horace Walpole called it, after the fairy tale of the three princes of Serendip, the former name for Ceylon. It happened just like this when we started trying to investigate Graves.

Our first expedition was in February 1969. I had been ill in hospital and wanted a few days away, so it was the perfect excuse to fly to Dublin. The snow started falling outside as we booked into the old Hibernian Hotel in Kildare Street, but there was a brisk fire burning in the hall and next day it was only a few steps to the Royal College of Physicians where we were made welcome in the library whose door is flanked by a splendid bust of Graves. Downstairs there was a statue of him standing very appropriately next to one of his great friends William Stokes. There was also a portrait, for he had been their President from 1843 to 1844. We read all we could find about him in the library. Next day we walked to the Royal College of Surgeons *in* Ireland (it is interesting that tradition makes it 'in' and not 'of,' where their library has much that bears upon Graves.

Armed with all this information we next hired a car and set off in search of local colour and drove to Limerick near which city the founder of the Irish branch of the Graves family had been given his lands by Cromwell. Limerick itself is a charming city and after tea we set off for the tiny village of Ardagh hoping to find a church and tombstones with clues to those early settlers. This was our first mistake because there are two Ardaghs in Eire, the other being in Co. Longford where we should have gone because Graves' father had been appointed dean there. In fact the church we found was newly built and Roman Catholic, but a drink in a nearby bar provided the whereabouts of a little Protestant church and cemetery about a mile up a narrow lane. The church was locked, there were a few gravestones and they were unkempt–the only one of interest was of an Australian from Sydney buried there in the nineteenth century. We had a good dinner and a quiet night in the hotel in Adare and set off early to shoot our last bolt by visiting Bunclody in the southeast of Ireland where we had been told that the Robertson family, descendants of Graves, now lived. It is a lovely drive through Tipperary to Cashell, with its castle on the rock and Archbishop's palace, to Kilkenny and so to Bunclody on the banks of the river Slaney. Nearby is the village of Clonegal, where we drove up a winding drive to Huntingdon Castle, an imposing old seventeenth century building with walls six feet thick.

Graves' descendants provide first breakthrough

We pulled the knob beside the door and heard the bell echoing down the stone flagged hall. Soon we were being greeted by Mr and Mrs Derek Robertson and their four children, all of whom were being educated at home. The castle was set in an estate of 150 acres of farmland and woods with birds everywhere and we felt quite at

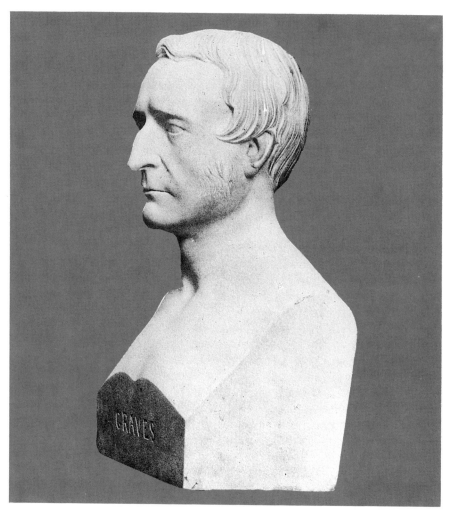

Bust of Graves by the Irish sculptor Hogan. It stands at the entrance to the Library of the Royal College of Physicians of Ireland in Kildare Street, Dublin. By courtesy of the Wellcome Museum, London.

home with the Welsh pony Taffy. Mr Robertson's grandmother had been Florence Graves, the youngest daughter of the great Dr Graves; she was twelve years younger than the other Graves children, due it was thought in the family to a marital rift which had been eventually resolved.

Our host could not have been more considerate nor more helpful and soon we were sitting at an old refectory table in the dining room; I was placed opposite the portrait of Florence who, it is said, burnt many of her father's letters because they would bring discredit on the family. Then we noticed a rustling noise coming from the direction of the great chimney breast whereupon two little curtains parted and out of the fireplace appeared a maid stooping and pushing a tea trolley, an entry for all the world like that of Father Christmas, made possible by the removal of the wall into the kitchen. The delicious sandwiches were filled with chives and sorrel from the garden and the bread was home baked using wholemeal flour made from wheat grown on the estate.

We were then conducted on a tour of the house, first to the old chapel, parts of which had now been rededicated to many religions other than Christianity; Muslim, Buddhist, Hindu, Osiris, and some which we did not understand. Our host had originally been a priest in the Anglican Church but was no longer practising its rites. Then we climbed upstairs where we entered a wonderful library lined with books and here was our first breakthrough. A little volume entitled *Some Notes on the Graves Family* by Hercules Henry Graves Macdonnell of Robyplace, Kingstown, dated March

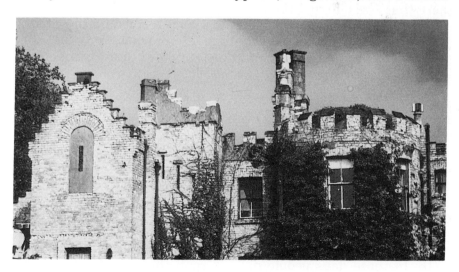

Huntingdon Castle, Clonegal, Co. Carlow.

1889 and printed for private circulation only. In its twenty two pages we found the whole history of the Graves family from the time of King John down through the English and Irish branches to the latter part of the nineteenth century. But more was to follow for Mr Robertson persuaded one of his daughters to climb up into the old lumber room and she returned hauling a very aged trunk. In it was a fascinating manuscript exercise book, the cover inscribed as follows:

Stemmata of
Nora Kathleen Parsons
who on Oct 15 1912
intermarried with
Manning Durdin Robertson
whose ancestors are given in the
Stemmata of Robertson and Durdin

Before we left Huntingdon Castle and the hospitable Robertsons we were presented with a little book of some 180 pages published in Dublin in 1960. It was entitled *Crowned Harp* and was written by Nora Robertson, daughter of Florence Graves and thus a granddaughter of Graves. It is a delightful and light hearted but shrewd account of the social and political history of Ireland in the early years of this century as seen through the eyes of a vivacious young woman brought up in a garrison in Ireland and later in England and in India. Finally her parents moved to Government House, Cork, as her father was appointed the General Commanding and it was from there that she married the architect, Manning Robertson, to become mistress of Huntingdon Castle. She is a splendid raconteur, always full of fun and delightfully irreverent, what a pity that she did not live a hundred years earlier to record the life and times of her illustrious grandfather.

Family roots in England
Back in England we read and reread the genealogy of the Graves family and the extraordinary succession of distinguished individuals; admirals, generals, governors and divines helped to explain why the doctor had been such an outstanding character. In addition, one of his forbears had been an antiquary and he claimed that the first member of the family whom he had been able to trace was one John de Grevis in King John's reign. His son Hugh and grandson William used the same spelling but the third in line styled himself Gyles del Greves who with his wife Lettice was living in 1316. In those days people did not spell their names with that constancy which we now expect and it was not long before Greves was corrupted to Graves and it was one Richard Graves who in 1656 bought the manor house in the village of Mickleton and founded that branch of the family in which we are interested.

Serendipity came to our aid once again. Holidaying in Cyprus we met the owner of Kiftsgate House, famous for its fine gardens and the home of the Kiftsgate rose. It almost adjoins the village of Mickleton and when we accepted an invitation to lunch we were introduced to the local general practitioner, Dr Olliff who, with his doctor wife, was a fount of knowledge on the village and its history and in addition, provided many excellent photographs. The last of the Graves family had only recently died and the manor house has now been divided into a number of homes.

The village church, dedicated to St Leonard, is well worth a visit since it is rich in historical monuments. It used to be the custom when the lord of the manor died, that his coat of arms, painted on a square wooden hatchment, was hung outside the house. In due course it was placed in the church and there is a fine collection of these hatchments at Mickleton. They hang on the north wall of the chancel and it is possible to deduce from them how from time to time the Graves family changed their motto: starting with *Superna Quarite* (seek those things which are above) it later became *Graves disce mores* thus punning on the family name (be concerned in Grave matters) and thirdly *Aquila non captat musces* (an eagle does not catch flies). Admiral Lord Graves, who was descended from the Northern Ireland branch of the family, was so enamoured of the

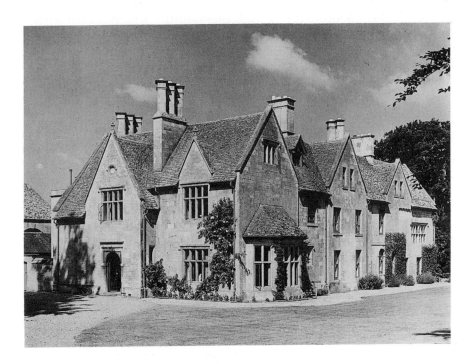

Mickleton House.

latter motto that he adopted it when he was ennobled. At the eastern end of the north wall there is a splendid memorial tablet by a local and talented sculptor, Edward Woodward, which commemorates many of the Graves family and is decorated with their coats of arms in colour.

Richard Graves, who was born in 1610, was a bencher of Lincoln's Inn and also became Clerk of the Peace and Receiver General for the county of Middlesex under Cromwell, of whom he seems to have been a personal friend. He purchased Mickleton Manor in which to reside in the year 1656, as well as the adjoining manors of Aston and Weston and the Royalty of Kiftsgate Hundred in which these manors are sited. The family succession was safe in his hands because he had six sons and nine daughters by his first wife and four daughters by his second marriage. He was a very short man with a fiery temper so that Cromwell used to say of him "Little pot, soon hot". His son Maurice married an admiral's daughter and their son Richard (always a favourite Christian name in the Graves family) is splendidly recorded in the church by a fine monument with a long Latin inscription setting forth his literary attainments, he was well known as the 'antiquary'. This Richard also had a son he called Richard, who was not only an author but a poet and in addition he wrote a novel *The Spiritual Quixote,* a satire on the Methodist Church which in his time was just beginning its spectacular rise to popularity. A book incidentally which is still obtainable. What is more, he erected a rather beautiful white memorial urn to his boyhood girl friend, Utrecia Smith, the curate's daughter, whom he wanted to marry, but for 'prudential reasons' did not; she poor girl died shortly afterwards of smallpox. The memorial now hides discreetly hidden behind the altar in the north chancel.

The move to Ireland
Now the Richard Graves who bought Mickleton Manor in 1656 had a younger brother William who also was a friend of Cromwell. William clearly had influence with the Protector and was sent to Ireland in 1650 as colonel of a horse regiment in the Parliamentary Army. He already had some standing in the army for he had a command at the siege of Bristol and was entrusted with the care of King Charles' person when he was taken from the camp of the Scots at Newcastle to Holmby House. It is difficult to write of Cromwell without taking sides because his character was such a strange mixture of religious fanaticism and sound commonsense. On the one hand he believed that everything he did was directed by God, yet he then proceeded to some unforgivable acts of cruelty and destruction. On the other hand he was a good son, husband and father with a genuine love of scholarship and music. Above all he was a leader with 'wonderful understanding in the natures and

humours of men'. But he certainly never understood Ireland nor the Irish. The uprising of 1641 which saw the death of so many Protestants ended up with the Government only holding a token area around Dublin, the Pale as it was called. Then Cromwell's men moved in and destroyed Ormonde's army, Irish and English, not forgetting many Roman Catholic priests. The conquest completed, something approaching half the country was handed over to English settlers. The wound thus caused has never healed soundly.

William Graves received a grant of land in county Kilkenny around Ballymack and Burnchurch and though he settled on his new Irish estate he remained both shrewd and far-seeing. He realised it could not be long before the end of the Parliamentary Government and the inevitable Restoration of the Monarchy, so he prudently sold his lands to a major in his regiment and returned to England with two of his sons. However he left two other sons behind and one of these, Henry, settled in the south near Limerick, some fifty miles to the west of the old home. The other brother went north and started an equally distinguished Anglo-Irish line of the family; one of his descendants was the Admiral Graves who so covered himself with distinction at the Glorious First of June under Lord Howe that he was created, there and then, an Irish peer—Baron Graves of Gravesend in the county of Londonderry.

Here however we are mainly concerned with Henry because it is from his family that our Dr Graves was descended. Henry had been born in 1652 and eventually settled in Graybridge near Limerick. The local folk nicknamed him 'Claymore' or 'Harry of the Long Sword' because when ever he went out he carried a huge sword to defend himself from the 'Irish Papists', he even went to the length of wearing it when he went to church in Croom which was his nearby town. In 1682 he had a son who was Christened John and later became a sheriff of the city of Limerick; his name is recorded on a plaque of a house in Bridge Street built by the corporation. John Graves had two sons and the eldest was appointed vicar of Kilfinnan and later rector of Mitchelstown. Of his five children the youngest was yet another Richard, born in 1763, and he was the father of our Dr Graves.

Graves' Parents

Over the centuries there have been many scholars in the family and Graves' father was one of these; having entered Trinity College Dublin he was made a Fellow at the unusually young age of twenty three. He was a theologian and is still remembered for his major work on the Pentateuch, that is the first five books of the Old Testament. Indeed, in old age the rest of the family used to refer to him as Pentateuch Graves! After a great deal of searching I was recently able to have a look at these lectures which were edited and published in four volumes by his eldest son, also called Richard, who was in turn a distinguished divine. The first volume was entirely given over to a memorial notice about the lecturer, who was of course his father, and the three remaining volumes contain the lectures. They were in fact sermons given as a result of the Donellan Legacy to Trinity and had to be delivered after morning service on Sundays in the College chapel. Those who attended were for the most part theology students who looked on the sermons as part of their degree course. I must add, in the interests of accuracy, that in fact the learned professor only discussed four of the Old Testament books and gave copious reasons why the book of Genesis was not germane to his thesis.

Graves' father certainly had a brilliant career at Trinity. So many of the Graves have been splendid scholars, divines or both and this one distinguished himself in classics, history, oratory and poetry. He graduated Master of Arts in 1787 and then took deacon's and priest's holy orders. When he was still only twenty-four he surreptitiously married his professor's daughter, Eliza Drought, and for the rest of a long life excelled at teaching and preaching. Twelve years later, in 1799, he was made a Senior Fellow and given the title of Professor of Oratory; then in 1814 he suceeded his father-in-law as Regius Professor of Divinity. He admitted in later life that he loved above all teaching the children at Sunday School at St Michael's Church in Dublin. He must have been successful, for it is recorded that children came from far and wide to hear him and eventually he had to give his talks on two days of the week, one for boys and one for girls. It is also recorded by his son that as a young man he combined his duties at Trinity with those of curate to a parish church and had the reputation of preaching the best sermons in the city. There can be little doubt that some of these spellbinding skills were inherited by his doctor son or perhaps they were acquired by sitting in the family pew on Sundays, for Graves was famous all his life for his powers of holding an audience.

Just to complete the story of Graves' parents, his mother Eliza whom his father had had to marry surreptitiously in case he lost his Fellowship, was a devoted wife and companion in everything her husband did until she died of a stroke in 1827. It was to recover from this loss that Graves' father spent a holiday in Keswick in the Lake District and there became friendly with the poet Southey. However a stroke brought his visit to an end and he died soon afterwards in Dublin at the age of 86.

Thus from the genetic point of view, Graves had a most promising background, his father was a Regius Professor of Divinity at Trinity, his mother the daughter of yet another professor. In addition, he grew up in a most happy and secure home with nine brothers and sisters. Finally he had great application and a positive zest for hard work.

Chapter 3

Growing Up

Graves was a fortunate child for he grew up in a happy home in Holles Street, near Trinity College, Dublin, surrounded by lots of brothers and sisters, something which was fairly common in Queen Victoria's reign and is so rare today. He was the seventh of ten children but in those days of poor life expectancy families were often large, and the Graves were no exception. His father was a Professor of Divinity at Trinity, his mother a professor's daughter and when the children went to school they were reckoned by all to be good scholars.

When one reads about life in Regency and early Victorian times there is a strong impression that authoritarianism pervaded the family structure and certainly Victorian divines appear to have been made of much sterner stuff than their latter-day equivalents. I have the distinct feeling that it was a very heavy and respectful atmosphere in the family home in Holles Street, Dublin, in which young Graves grew up—but a happy one. Discipline and contentment so often go hand in hand. Where there are many young brothers and sisters there is plenty of companionship and great opportunities for fun together. In addition to this, in a large family, children tend to educate each other in so many ways and soon develop close and lasting bonds of fellowship. Robert was born in 1796 and his great friend was his brother Hercules, two years his senior; the two boys were devoted to each other and their careers for many years ran parallel. The unusual Christian name of Hercules was inherited from a Huguenot ancestor on his mother's side.

Oscar Wilde's uncle prepares Graves for University entrance

Graves, like his brothers and sisters, started his education at the Downpatrick Diocesan School where he was a good pupil. In those days it was not unusual to have a private tutor for those in their teens, especially when they were to be prepared for university entrance, and certainly all the Graves boys were so destined. Both Hercules and Robert were taught by the Revd Ralph Wilde. Tutors play such an important role in the impressionable teenage years, both in developing character as well as intellect that it is important to see what kind of man was chosen as the young Graves' mentor. The Revd Wilde had the reputation in Dublin of being an eminent scholar, which indeed he had been at Trinity. He came from a family which produced some distinguished scions and a look at their achievements throws more light on the subject.

It is I believe possible to draw a parallel between the great emigration of the Irish to America in the nineteenth century and that of the English to Ireland in the seventeenth and eighteenth. The Irish have thrived in the USA, bringing their own distinctive characteristics, and their descendants have enriched every walk of life from the White House to the farming communities of the middle west. In different but not dissimilar manner the English went to Ireland and the resultant Anglo-Irish descendants have likewise infused strength into most walks of life from the universities to the armed forces and to commerce. Indeed it has often been pointed out that their offspring have in many cases become much more Irish in outlook than the indigenous Celt. The Wildes are a good example; Ralph Wilde was a builder in Walsingham near Durham in the northeast of England and he was attracted by the great expansion of house building which took place in Dublin in Georgian times, so he settled there with his family. He prospered and one of his sons, also called Ralph, went to Connaught and became agent for Lord Mount Sandford at Castlerea. He married Margaret O'Flynn who was the daughter of an ancient Irish family and they had three sons. One of them became a surgeon who lived at Number 1 Merrion Square and the other was Ralph who was ordained priest and was widely known for his learning, winning the Berkeley Gold Medal for Greek at Trinity, and coached many prominent young men who would later achieve fame in their own right. Incidentally the surgeon had two sons one of whom was none other than the playwright Oscar Wilde. Thus the tutor whom the Graves family employed was an uncle of Oscar Wilde.

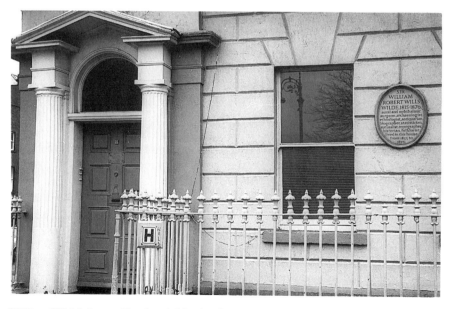

William Wilde's house, Number 1, Merrion Square.

There can be no doubt that the reverend doctor was an excellent teacher and, in addition, coach for the examinations, for first he tutored young Hercules who then passed into Trinity with a scholarship and was head of all the entries. As an undergraduate, Hercules continued to excel, so he must have had real talent in his own right and when he finally graduated, he was the one to be awarded the gold medal at the top of the honours list. Some two years later young Robert having also been coached by Wilde similarly passed into Trinity at the top of the entry list and his subsequent career at this establishment merits a chapter to itself.

Hercules, unfortunately, was always said to be delicate and all too often in Victorian times the word 'delicate' was really a euphemism for having pulmonary tuberculosis, although at that time the true nature of the disease and the tubercle bacillus which causes it, had yet to be discovered. No doubt the long hours that he spent studying at his desk and in the library at Trinity, together with the damp Irish climate, were aggravating factors. Thus it was that in 1817 the ailing Hercules, accompanied by his elder brother Richard and younger sister Anna, set off for the South of France, hoping that the warmer climate of Provence would bring about a cure. Clearly the family were quite well to do at this time to be able to afford such an expense. Sadly Hercules died before the end of the year and in the little Protestant section of the mainly Roman Catholic cemetery at Aix-en-Provence there is a headstone which states that he died on November 6th 1817. Graves was later to visit the grave during his travels in Europe and was very moved by the experience.

Graves' other siblings
What of Graves' other eight brothers and sisters? The best way to understand the family as a whole is to look at the diagram of the family tree. It has been transcribed from Nora Parsons' hand written stemmata. Stemma, the Latin word for a wreath, has by long usage come to mean family tree, and since she traced the pedigree of many branches of her ancestors she inscribed the cover of her exercise book with the plural, stemmata!

The picture that now emerges of the family of Richard and Eliza Graves is one that is fairly representative of the nineteenth century when infant mortality was high compared to present day standards and when adults, especially in the lower age bracket, regularly succumbed to tuberculosis. William Osler, ninety years ago, still referred to it as the 'universal scourge of the human race'. However, the Graves came of sturdy stock and many of them lived well into their eighties. It still appears to me a daunting prospect, having ten children in thirteen years; Eliza must have been a very busy person. In those days there would of course have been a small army of servants working in the home: housekeeper, cook, maids and at least one nurserymaid.

Very Revd Richard Graves b 1 Oct 1763, d 31 Mar 1829
Dean of Ardagh. Fellow of Trinity College Dublin. Regius Professor of Divinity
m Aug 1 1787 Eliza Mary Drought d Mar 22 1827.
Daughter of Professor of Divinity James Drought TCD.
later Dean of Ardagh and Regius Professor

John. James. Richard. Eliza. Jane. Hercules. Robert. Anna. Harriet. Bella

1. John Graves, b 1788, d young.
2. James Drought Graves, b Jan 1790, d aged 4.
3. Richard Hastings Graves (Revd), b 10 Jan 1791, d Dec 1877, Life in NDB.
4. Eliza Graves, b Mar 1792, m1 Revd Thomas Meredith Drew, Fellow TCD,
   m2 Revd James Burton.
5. Jane Graves, b Mar 1793, m Jan 26 1810 Richard Macdonnell,
   Fellow TCD.
6. Hercules Henry Graves, b Oct 14 1794, d Nov 6 1817.
7. Robert James Graves, MD, FRS, b Mar 28 1796, d Mar 20 1853.
8. Anna Graves, b Mar 1798, d 1864, m1 Edward Johnson, m2 John Mayne.
9. Harriet Graves, b Mar 1800, d Apr 27 1855, m Matthew Brinkley.
10. Arabella Graves, b Mar 1801, d May 23 1879, unmarried.

Graves' immediate family, from Nora Parsons' stemmata.

Apart from his great friend Hercules, Graves' nine brothers and sisters seem rarely to have crossed his path in his subsequent life, certainly he does not mention them in what correspondence has survived, so let us look at them quite briefly here. First of all there was John Graves (1788) who died soon after birth, then James Drought Graves (1790) who was usually referred to in the family as the eldest because the first born had died so young. James died from an acute attack of scarlet fever when he was only four years old. Such a cause of death in this country is almost unheard of today, not only because treatment is now greatly improved because of the introduction of antibiotics, which is undoubtedly true, but because the disease has over the years lost its sting. Next came Richard (1791), the most popular Christian name with the Graves for many generations. He was another of the intellectual members of the family and lived to a great age, 86. He took holy orders and became distinguished enough to find a place in the Dictionary of National Biography.

Then there was Eliza (1792) who married first the Revd Thomas Meredith who was a Fellow of Trinity College and after he died in 1819 she remarried in 1824 another rector, James Burton. Jane

Graves (1793) married at seventeen a Fellow of Trinity College who was a don there, his name was Richard Macdonnell and he in due course became Provost of Trinity, but he died in 1867 and she outlived him for fifteen years. Of their nine children one was a Governor of many colonies from South Australia to Hong Kong, another was a major general and a third, Judge of the Westminster County Court.

Finally the three children who were younger than Graves were all girls. First was Anna (1798) who married twice and all her family had something to do with the legal profession, either becoming lawyers or barristers or marrying them. The ninth child was Harriet (1800) who married Matthew Brinkley, son of the Astronomer Royal of Ireland who was later Bishop of Cloyne, one of their sons was a distinguished professor in Japan. Last but by no means least was Arabella (1801) who died unmarried in Dublin in 1879. She was known to the next generation of Graves children as the formidable Aunt Bella. This then, is the complete list of Graves' brothers and sisters, and it is remarkable what a distinguished group of Victorians they grew up to be.

Great Aunt Bella as the grandchildren called her was considered 'a dreadful tartar'. Indeed, she used to force the younger members of the family to learn a hymn each week and repeat it to her under penalty of hell fire for failure. In *Crowned Harp,* the light hearted autobiography of her early life in India and later in Ireland before Irish independence, Nora Robertson tells one of the family stories about her mother, Florence, Graves' youngest child, who was born long after the rest of the family. It seems that once young Flo's elder brother William, a fast young man, taught her a new verse, gave her a shilling and told her to repeat these lines in her hymn to Aunt Bella and then he waited at the keyhole for the inevitable explosion. Poor Little Flo did her bit:
> "Damn your eyes, if ever you tries
> to rob a poor man of his beer".

Great Aunt Bella could not trust hell to deal with such enormity, Little Flo got a severe whacking on earth. William, a thoroughly nasty piece of work, just ran off and left her to her fate, says Nora Robertson.

An atmosphere of social change
Certainly the years during which the young Graves grew up in Dublin saw far reaching changes in that city and not only there, for across the water in England and France the old order was being overthrown. In France the Revolution virtually exploded with the storming of the Bastille on July 14th 1789 and in October the mob marched on Versailles and brought the French King and the Royal

Family back to Paris. Sweeping changes were made in the constitution, Louis XVI was executed in 1793 and not until July 1794 was the Reign of Terror ended and Robespierre beheaded. It was the young Napoleon Bonaparte who put down the insurrection in Paris in October the following year and by the time that young Graves was first seeing the light of day in Dublin in 1796, Bonaparte was winning his early battles in Northern Italy.

Chapter 4

Trinity College Dublin
Europe in Turmoil

The Trinity College at which Graves presented himself looked very much the same as it does today. Trinity College, or the University of Dublin as it was originally known, was founded by Queen Elizabeth I in 1592 on the site of a monastery dispossessed fifty years earlier by Henry VIII. It was originally 'near Dublin', between the houses and the sea, until it was engulfed by the expanding city. Situated on a forty acre site in what is now the centre of Dublin it has suceeded in cloistering itself, so that as you enter you seem to pass into another world which has a splendid feeling of ancient seclusion. What first strikes the visitor is the imposing Palladian façade which was built in 1759 and is still graced by two fine statues of Goldsmith and Burke. The first quadrangle or Parliament Square contains the chapel with its Corinthian portico and the public theatre, which is an examination hall containing portraits of Queen Elizabeth and Bishop Berkeley. The central square has a lovely campanile tower that was added in 1853, and the library built between 1712 and 1732 houses one of the most outstanding collections of books in the British Isles or indeed anywhere in the world. It contains many manuscripts and, always on view, the famous book of Kells with its exquisitely decorated manuscript text of the Gospels.

We have to remember that at the time that Graves was studying at Trinity this was the only university in Dublin. Though greatly dominated by the Protestant community, it was loyally Irish, and both staff and administration often held views opposed to those of the government in London. The staff were for the most part descendants of the English and Scots who had made Ireland their home over the centuries, but the great reputation which Trinity had gained in the world of learning constantly attracted fresh blood from other centres in the English speaking countries. A good example is the famous Cambridge mathematician and wrangler Brinkley, who came from Woodbridge in Suffolk and was appointed Professor of Mathematics; eventually he became Astronomer Royal in Ireland and his daughter married Graves. Although unfortunately she died a year later, the two families were to be linked again in the next generation. Scholars came from all over the world to study at Trinity as indeed they are still doing to this day. It is always a joy to visit Trinity because the fabric of the place is so lovingly maintained.

An excellent appreciation of the importance of Trinity, or as it is affectionately called today, TCD, is provided by the social historian GM Trevelyan in his foreword to Maxwell's *History of Trinity College Dublin:* "A unique institution", he says "which for three and a half centuries has embraced so much of what was best, greatest and happiest in the chequered career of Ireland. The proportion of famous Irish names upon its rolls is wonderful—names of poets, satirists, novelists, orators, scientists, historians, men of learning in every branch of study, publicists and politicians of every party. What other college, I had almost said what other university, could show a nobler roll? One is struck by the liberality of Trinity College in days when little else in Ireland was liberal. Furthermore, in the eighteenth century, when almost all other endowed and established institutions in the British Isles were struck with paralysis, when Oxford and Cambridge declined shamefully in numbers, in enterprise and reputation, the Alma Mater of Edmund Burke was flourishing and adorning herself with new buildings. The character and achievement of Trinity, Dublin has been due to Irishmen."

Other seats of learning

It was not until 1854 that John Henry Newman, later to be made Cardinal, went to Dublin at the request of the Irish Bishops to be Rector of a newly established Catholic University; Trinity was a Protestant stronghold in what was very largely a Catholic city. The major result of this appointment was a series of lectures which were later published in a volume entitled *The Idea of a University,* a work that is still often quoted today. But conditions were not favourable for Newman to set up such a new university at that time and he retired after four years to England where he founded a school in association with the Birmingham Oratory. He was not made a Cardinal until 1879. Eventually the Roman Catholic community did set up a university which they called the National University of Ireland, much of it was situated originally at the corner of St Stephen's Green on the site of the old International Exhibition of 1865. Some of the faculties have now moved to a more spacious site further from the centre of the city at Elm Park on the road to the south.

Before the days of partition the Queens University of Ireland had important colleges, as they were called at that time, in Belfast, Cork and Galway and these all survive to this day. Having grown enormously, each has become an independent university in its own right. Today the old rivalry between the essentially Roman Catholic National University of Ireland and the basically Protestant Trinity College, Dublin is muted. No longer is it necessary to profess a certain religion in order to obtain a degree at either place. There is a sharing of resources and intermingling of the intellectual skills, greatly accelerated in the last twenty years by the medical faculties with their free interchange of students, together with recognition of each other's examinations and degrees. Despite all this, one is never allowed to forget that Ireland is still a land where religion plays a powerful part in the social and academic patterns of society and continues to be divisive—especially north of the border.

The splendour of Trinity College and Dublin in Graves' days
The eighteenth century was certainly the period of Trinity College's palmy days and Dublin in those days was riding high; James Morton wrote "Dublin is the second city in His Britannic Majesty's Dominions, and may rank with the very finest cities of Europe for extent, magnificence and commerce". The present day visitor to Dublin, and I count myself fortunate to be one of these, cannot fail to be impressed and charmed by the spaciousness of the squares and boulevards which are reminiscent in their elegant proportions of Paris and Vienna and are at last, I am glad to see, being restored to some of their former glory. Unfortunately many beautiful Georgian façades have disappeared as a result of the speculative builders and developers moving in, especially in the 1950s and 1960s. Those decades have left a miserable architectural legacy to be seen in many of our cities—not least in London.

In the 1780s and 1790s the Provost of Trinity was John Hely-Hutchison. He had been an undistinguished graduate of Trinity by any standards and certainly if judged by those of the Graves' family, but he later became a barrister and a member of Parliament and finally, when Secretary of State in the Irish Parliament, he obtained by skilfull influence the title of Provost of Trinity. He is still remembered for the manner in which he enlarged the Provost's house to accommodate his growing family and their many servants; it has a glorious staircase and beautifully proportioned rooms. More importantly however he is also remembered for his startling innovation in those days of establishing Chairs in modern languages, since at that time the main accent of the curriculum was on Latin, Greek, theology and law. Science and the medical faculty were poor relations. He was certainly an outstanding Provost and a liberal one, in an establishment which at that time was only liberal in respect of learning for it still clung to its ancient and bigotted anti-catholicism when it came to religion. He regarded as disgraceful the obnoxious oaths which were imposed on Catholics in Trinity before admission to their degrees. Indeed before he died in 1794 he was successful in having these tests abolished. When Edmund Burke, who had graduated there in 1747, was brought back in 1790 to receive an honorary LL D from his old Alma Mater he declaimed with his customary eloquence, which in many ways is typical of that era, that "the University was highly generous in accepting with so much indulgence the product of its own gift".

Graves excelled in his studies and extra-curricular activities

The foundations of Graves' extraordinary scholarship which he so often demonstrated later in both lecturing and writing throughout his professional life, were clearly laid down at this time. He entered for his studies at Trinity under Dr Meredith and was afterwards transferred to Dr Elrington. His syllabus included both science and classics and having obtained first place in a particularly large July entrance he proceeded to maintain the same pre-eminent place throughout his whole course, so Sir William Wilde tells us, and with two exceptions he received the 'first premium' and also certificates in both science and classics at every examination up to his so-called 'fellow commoners degree'. Thus we find young Graves in 1815 passing out from Trinity with his Bachelor of Arts degree, and receiving the gold medal, the highest award obtainable by students of Trinity at that time, just as elder brothers Richard and subsequently, Hercules, had done before him.

Graves had great vitality and such an active and enquiring mind that he joined in many of the extra-curricular activities and became a member of a variety of student societies. Students have always avidly discussed current events and at that time they were undoubtedly witnessing the reshaping of the old regime in Europe. In 1815 Wellington and Blucher won the battle of Waterloo and the subsequent Congress of Vienna changed the map of Europe and thus marked the end of an era. Graves was thrilled by the discussions in the College Historical Society, founded by Burke in his student days as the 'Historical Club'; it has probably witnessed more eloquence than any other debating forum in Europe. We know from a number of eye witnesses that Graves schooled himself to be a brilliant lecturer and what better training ground can there be anywhere in the whole world than a debating society in Dublin. As a boy young Graves had sat at his father's feet Sunday after Sunday listening to one of the city's outstanding preachers who was also Professor of Oratory at Trinity and now the College Historical Society's meetings showed him how to use these skills in other fields. He could not have had a better grounding nor proved a more receptive pupil.

Political changes causing turbulence in Ireland and throughout Europe

Historians sometimes draw the inference that certain periods in time are peculiarly suited to the appearance of particularly gifted individuals and the Renaissance is indeed a good example of this, but in the sciences, and especially the medical sciences, the converse can be true and I believe that often it can be the arrival on the scene of a single brilliant or original intellect that leads to the development of a new climate of opinion and endeavour. Certainly the years in which Graves grew up and graduated at Trinity were singularly inauspicious in the scientific and especially the medical field. Stokes, his outstanding pupil and later friend and colleague, looking back on the period from 1800 to 1821 described it as "characterised rather by a kind of mental collapse than by activity, such a result" he went on to say "might be naturally expected, when the political changes which the country had undergone are considered". The political history of Ireland is certainly a chequered one and the first quarter of the nineteenth century was no exception.

In 1805 the British fleet under the greatest commander she has known, Lord Nelson, decisively defeated the French and Spanish navies at Trafalgar and Napoleon turned from his plan to invade England, withdrew his troops from Boulogne and marched to the Danube. In less than two months he was in Vienna and had defeated the Emperors of Austria and Russia at Austerlitz. In England, Pitt as Prime Minister had guided the Act of Union with Ireland through Parliament. In the North of Ireland particularly, the Protestants and Catholics were at each other's throats and in Ulster the Protestants founded the Orange Society to protect their interests.

In the South of Ireland, Wolfe Tone was looking to France for support and the Parliament in Dublin was utterly corrupt. Clearly Pitt had cherished hopes that the Bill of Union between Ireland and England might succeed as had the previous Union of England with Scotland; but the stumbling block with the Irish proved to be as always, Roman Catholicism. On top of all this, George III, the Farmer King, refused his royal assent. Pitt resigned and as a result, catholic emancipation was delayed for almost thirty years. Meanwhile the Act of Union was carried through the Irish Parliament by means of patronage and bribery and the Chamber in Westminster absorbed the Irish Members. Winston Churchill, in his *Short History of the English Speaking Peoples,* put it in his typically succinct way: "Bitter fruits were to follow" and still they do today, 180 years later.

Graves aquires a love of learning that becomes the basis of his postgraduate career

Despite all this turbulent background in Ireland and indeed in Europe as a whole, young Graves seems to have had a wonderfully successful and apparently happy three years at Trinity. It was to prove of inestimable benefit to him during the rest of his life, for he acquired a solid base of scholarship and a real love of learning. He also obtained an excellent knowledge of Latin, always an asset for a doctor, since it forms the basis for so many medical terms. In addition he developed a genuine love of classical literature from Virgil to Horace both of whom he enjoyed quoting for the rest of his life. Above all he learnt how to learn, a matter of major import, because his medical education both undergraduate and postgraduate was to occupy the next six years of his life. The modern philosophy of our educators in medicine is that postgraduate medical education takes two forms. The first is now called higher medical training and can last anything from four to six years. During this period the doctor holds various registrar posts which rotate between his university or teaching hospital and the hurly burly of practice in a district hospital, his work being monitored throughout. Eventually he becomes a senior registrar and when he has satisfied the requirements of the Royal Colleges he is said to be 'accredited' and can then apply for a consultant post. In addition to this, most of us would agree today with the philosophy that postgraduate medical education starts immediately the day after the young doctor qualifies and continues until final retirement, and it is this later phase of updating medical knowledge which constitutes the second phase of postgraduate study. In no other way can the present day doctor hope to keep abreast of current advances—indeed if he fails to do this today there is the ever present threat of medical litigation and although in Britain this has reached nowhere near the level seen in the USA, it escalates yearly.

In Graves' day there were no rules about postgraduate training, any young man (and women were not then accepted into the medical profession) as soon as he had obtained a medical degree or diploma could start to practice. But Graves planned, as we shall see, a thorough grounding in postgraduate study and thereafter never ceased studying throughout his professional life.

Chapter 5

Medical School

The young Graves having now distinguished himself by obtaining the gold medal in his BA degree had to choose by which method he would proceed to a medical qualification. There were three avenues open to him in Dublin at that time and his eventual standing among his fellow doctors might well depend on which path he took. The easiest course would be to apply to one of the numerous private or chartered medical schools which in those days flourished in the city, many of their successful candidates passing in to the armed forces or emigrating—Ireland already had a reputation for exporting doctors. The second route, and one much favoured by the Trinity graduates of the day was to enrol in the medical school in Edinburgh which had a high standing in Europe and offered superior clinical instruction to Dublin or indeed any other centre in the British Isles. The third possibility, and the one which Graves in the event did opt for, was to enter the medical faculty at Trinity which of course he already knew well. The disadvantages of such a choice were that the clinical teaching would not be as good as in Edinburgh but to some extent this failing had recently been compensated for in Dublin with the opening of the new Sir Patrick Dun's Hospital, to which the Trinity men went for their bedside instruction instead of having to traipse all over the city to the numerous small hospitals which had previously catered for them. These were the days when medical students were said to 'walk the wards'. Accordingly, Graves signed on at Trinity for the three year course and had no difficulty in gaining acceptance since he had such an excellent previous record as a student and, in addition, his father was a professor at Trinity.

Studying medicine before the mid nineteenth century
The University of Dublin's original charter which was granted by Elizabeth I in 1597 empowered it to give medical degrees, but this privilege was not exercised until 1674. The medical school, or as it was known in the seventeenth century, the school of physic, required that its students first obtain a degree in the humanities, a term used to cover a general education in Latin, Greek and the arts. This requirement is still demanded first at the universities of Oxford and Cambridge and throughout the USA, but the degree of those eventually proceeding to a medical qualification for which most candidates opt today is more usually one in the natural sciences, especially physiology or anatomy rather than the arts. However, the great majority of the universities in the British Isles

including London, which has far and away the biggest number of medical students, now allow them to proceed directly to their medical course without any such preliminary education. From my own experience, both as student and teacher, I firmly believe that a first degree in the non-clinical field is much to be preferred, since the student acquires a broader base of learning, learns how to study without the strict discipline to which he has become accustomed at school and so approaches medicine as an althogether more mature individual. Most young men and women when they first arrive at university need to let off a lot of steam before they adjust to their new found freedom.

Eoin O'Brien, who is a cardiologist in Dublin and a distinguished medical historian, published in 1983 a life of Dr Dominic Corrigan who was a contemporary of Graves. Corrigan was eminent in his day not only as a physician with a special interest in diseases of the heart and blood vessels, but also he was very prominent in medical politics. Fortunately he seems never to have destroyed any of his papers, diplomas and correspondence and their discovery in a chest at the Royal College of Physicians of Ireland has provided us with a wonderful insight into every aspect of nineteenth century medicine in Dublin. From a study of these papers, O'Brien has been able to piece together a picture of medical education at the very time that Graves was in medical school. He is able to point out that there were very real advantages in taking the medical course at Trinity, not least that once the candidate obtained his final medical degree he was automatically made a licentiate of the Royal College of Physicians. This entitled him to call himself a physician and to practice as such in Dublin. Candidates from the private medical schools were not recognised by the College until they had submitted to a further examination.

Medical qualifications have always been much more complicated in the British Isles than anywhere else in the world. In practically every country overseas the sole degree that the doctor requires is the MD, but in England, Scotland and Ireland there is a far greater choice. First of all universities have the right to award medical degrees and their standard is regularly monitored by the General Medical Council or GMC. Second there is an independent body, the Society of Apothecaries who are also entitled to give a diploma which permits medical practice. Thirdly there are the Royal Colleges, of Physicians and of Surgeons who are the guardians of standards of clinical training and who award a series of diplomas: licentiate, member and fellow in ascending degree. A further source of confusion is that the Royal Colleges in London, Edinburgh, Glasgow and Dublin have minor variations between each other. It is salutary to remember that John Keats after a three year apprenticeship to a country doctor proceded to the United Hospitals of

Guy's and St Thomas' and on July 25th 1816 obtained his diploma to practice medicine following an examination at the Society of Apothecaries in Blackfriars, London.

In Dublin at the beginning of the nineteenth century there was a plethora of medical schools and Sir Charles Cameron, biographer and historian of the Royal College of Surgeons in Ireland gives a list of what he describes as the 'unchartered or private' establishments. Named for the founder or by their location they include:

1728 Brenn
1804 Crampton
1808 Jervis Street
1809 Kirby
1812 House of Industry Hospitals
1820 Moore Street
1821 Anatomy and Surgery School, Lower Ormond Quay
1822 Eccles Street
1824 Park Street. Graves amongst others was the founder. It closed in 1849
1821 Richmond Hospital. Also known as Carmichael

Graves' first year in the medical school was largely taken up learning what were for him the new disciplines of anatomy, physiology and chemistry, for his previous degree had been almost exclusively in the arts and he had only learnt a minimum of science. All medical students when they first enter the dissecting room of the anatomy department feel fairly mixed emotions at the sight of rows of human bodies laid out on the tables for their dissection. Certainly young Graves was in no way discouraged because he returned after completing the required tasks to study human anatomy in greater detail than was demanded by his examiners.

The influence of Robert Perceval
At that time the Professor of Chemistry at Trinity was a particularly distinguished man named Robert Perceval who was destined to have a profound influence in shaping the young Graves' interests and his character. He became not only teacher but a close friend and it was to Perceval that Graves addressed most of his letters when he travelled abroad, asking him to pass them on to his other friends after he had read them. Perceval was already a senior member of the faculty when Graves arrived. He was a relation of the Earls of Egremont which gave him considerable standing in the social life of the city and it was his cousin Spencer Perceval who in May 1812 while Prime Minister of England was shot dead as he entered the lobby of the Houses of Parliament. Robert Perceval was born in 1756 and studied both chemistry and medicine at Trinity. In 1785 he was elected the Foundation Professor of Chemistry and was responsible

for building the first ever laboratories in Trinity. In the following year the Government appointed him to be Inspector of Apothecaries and as a result he came to have a wide knowledge of the medical provisions in the country as a whole. The Irish Government had set up a kind of National Health Service with its nationwide series of dispensaries at each of which a medically qualified apothecary attended, thus providing medical care for those who could not afford to pay for the services of a private medical practitioner. These apothecaries were employed part time and miserably paid; in time their poor pay was to become a cause célèbre during the typhus and cholera epidemics.

Perceval realised that the outstanding need of the medical students at Trinity was a teaching hospital of their own where they could go and receive bedside instruction by clinicians appointed by the university and approved of by the Royal College of Physicians, because at that time they were still spending much of the day time travelling around Dublin to a multitude of small private hospitals. Since there was a suitable source of money available in the Sir Patrick Dun bequest he requested the university authorities to authorise such a plan. In doing so he immediately fell foul of the Professor of Botany, Edward Hill, who was similarly determined to use the bequest for a university physic garden. Professor Hill was in a strong position since he was both Professor of Physic as well as Professor of Botany, but Perceval employed all his considerable talents as a medical politician to win the battle. In these days of highly sophisticated pharmaceutical products, from penicillin to the cephalosporins with which to treat infection, and a multitude of other powerful agents like cortisone and the beta-blockers, it is difficult to remember that until fifty years ago almost all the remedies a doctor could use were of plant origin. Thus a century ago a large part of the curriculum of a medical student was taken up by botany and the study of plant products so that Professor Hill's desire for a university physic garden, as a teaching aid, was very reasonable. In the light of subsequent events Perceval's teaching hospital plan was undoubtedly correct, but I cannot help feeling a little sorry for Professor Hill. The upshot of this politico-academic battle was that Professor Hill lost the day and resigned the chair of physic; when you enter the hall of the Royal College of Physicians in Dublin you see hanging on the wall the portrait of a disappointed man.

It was on account of his falling under the spell of Perceval that Graves was for the rest of his professional life interested in the chemical interpretation of the mechanisms of living organisms both in health and disease. He would be described in these days as a biochemist manqué or perhaps better, a clinical pharmacologist, and Perceval himself might similarly be described as such. It was however in the study of anatomy that Graves showed interest far in excess of what was required at that time. Traditionally, physicians were not expected to have a very thorough knowledge of the subject, unlike those destined to be surgeons. Indeed in the early nineteenth century, surgeons were lumped together in the public's mind with barbers, periwig makers and apothecaries, whilst physicians, like lawyers and parsons, were looked on as gentlemen and when they called to visit the sick were admitted by the front door. But times were changing and the College of Surgeons petitioned the Crown in 1784 and obtained a Royal Charter which entitled them to be called the Royal College of Surgeons in Ireland in 1784 just six years after the surgeons in Edinburgh had done the very same thing. In 1810 the Irish College built a medical school immediately behind the main building on St Stephen's Green and it was in the dissecting rooms there that Graves pursued some additional knowledge of human anatomy which he was so keen to have. For the rest of his life Graves always maintained that a thorough grounding in anatomy was essential for a doctor and he was particularly fortunate in that his first teacher and the head of the anatomy department at Trinity was Professor James Macartney. He certainly exerted a profound influence on the young Graves and as he was such a talented and controversial figure at Trinity it is worth describing his background.

James Macartney head of anatomy

Macartney was born in Armagh in 1770 when, under the old Anglo-Irish rule, the Catholics had not yet been emancipated. Being a tall boy for his age, when only ten years old he was enrolled in Lord Charlemont's Volunteers and would recall with what delight he put on the splendid uniform which he was given. In later life he was to write "I was greatly flattered by the attention which I received from all who were interested in that armament. When Lord Charlemont and his family came into the country, attended by Grattan and other leaders of that time, I always went to them after dinner. The ladies kissed and carressed me, and Grattan on one occasion carried me round the room on his shoulder". "These were the days" wrote Macartney, perhaps distance had led to enchantment, "when Erin was great, glorious and free. The Catholics were not emancipated by law, but by what was much better, the sense of justice of the Protestants. They were taken into the volunteer companies, although subject to the penal statute of carrying arms. They then first enjoyed something like equality, and acquired the love of freedom".

He was an enthusiastic supporter of the United Irishmen and in 1792 formed a branch in his native town of Armagh. He went to work in his uncle's linen office in Newry and fell in love with Miss Elkenhead, but his first proposal of marriage was cut short by the untimely arrival of his uncle and later the young lady herself rejected his advances. So he gave up the idea of marriage and went home "where my attention was directed to surgery, not for any taste for the profession, but having sufferred the inconvenience of a compassionate disposition, which with me amounted to an infirmity, I thought surgery would harden my heart, as it did others. In this I have been disappointed".

Macartney went to Dublin in 1793 and entered the School of the Royal College of Surgeons and was apprenticed to Hartigan whom he was eventually to succeed as Professor of Anatomy. Again he fell in love, the infirmity is incurable, this time with the beautiful Miss Singer. "I might have proposed for her if she had not been so extraordinarily thin. From the thread paper figure she grew into one of the most bulky women I ever saw. How little people can tell what their wives may become in person, temper or principles". In anatomy he soon proved to be the outstanding pupil of his year, working inordinately hard, thus when he went home to Newry for the vacation he appeared so physically run down that Miss Elkenhead's sympathy was finally aroused and they were in due course married. He did not complete his studies in the College of Surgeons at Dublin but was lured to the famous anatomy school in Great Windmill Street in London, founded by William Hunter who was the leading obstetrician of his day—a bachelor who spent all his money and his working hours on practice and research and left a magnificent heritage to his old medical school in Glasgow. It was William who invited his young brother John Hunter to join him in teaching and research in the anatomy school which became the most famous in Europe under the brothers' reign. No wonder that the ambitious Macartney was attracted there. John Hunter is generally regarded as the father of the English school of surgical research. Meanwhile Macartney, at the same time that he demonstrated anatomy found time to pursue his clinical studies at Guy's, St Thomas' and St Bartholomew's; in those days the medical student literally 'walked the wards'. At St Bartholomew's Hospital in Smithfield his outstanding ability was noticed by Abernethy who appointed him demonstrator in anatomy and subsequently lecturer in comparative anatomy.

Always a fiery individual, Macartney was soon at loggerheads with his colleagues and had to resign his demonstratorship, but was able to retain his lectureship. He joined the army and was posted to the Isle of Wight whence he obtained leave each academic year to deliver his lectures in London, thus retaining his appointment as lecturer. In 1811 when he was 41, having already written some outstanding papers in the field of comparative anatomy and embryology, his labours were rewarded by election as a Fellow of the Royal Society and the same year he was posted with his regiment to

Ireland. A year later the regiment was disbanded in Dublin and, having visited St Andrew's University to obtain an MD, for he was not yet medically qualified, he was appointed to succeed Hartigan at Trinity in 1813 as Professor of Anatomy and Chirurgery. He was still only 43 and was to occupy the chair for the next twenty-four years, revitalising not only his own department of anatomy, but the rest of Trinity as well. He was indeed a turbulent spirit.

Macartney started by outlawing Latin as the language used in lectures and examinations, whereupon the King's professors reported this to the College of Physicians. The latter body decided that the King's professors should not be present at any examination for medical degrees at which any question might be put or any answer received in the English language. In addition they stipulated that the lectures at Sir Patrick Dun's Hospital and all the patients' case notes should be in the Latin tongue—despite all this Macartney eventually won the day. Latin was in general use by doctors and students in those days so that the patient should not understand what was being said, but by all accounts the Latin often sounded like the mumbo jumbo of a witch doctor. The same spirit of secrecy has in a lesser degree lasted right down to our own times with the writing of prescriptions in Latin, but quite recently plain English has replaced it in the UK.

Macartney was intellectually head and shoulders above his colleagues and his originality must have been due in no small part to some of the Hunter brothers' spirit of curiosity rubbing off on him during his years at the Great Windmill school of anatomy. He enjoyed having young Graves as a pupil at Trinity, with his sharp enquiring intellect and he encouraged him. Certainly Graves had a lifelong interest in comparative anatomy and embryology which had been fostered at this early period. Graves, like his teacher, also disapproved of the use of dog Latin at the bedside, it must have been a splendid cloak for ignorance, and later condemned it at his inaugural lecture to the students when he was appointed as physician to Sir Patrick Dun's Hospital. Here are the actual words he used when damning the practice: "When this information was conveyed, as it formerly was at Sir Patrick Dun's Hospital, in Latin, the student had to encounter another barrier to the acquisition of knowledge. I have called the language LATIN, in compliance with the generally conceived opinion concerning its nature". The replacement of dog Latin by English in medical teaching was certainly pioneered by Dublin and it is interesting to note that a similar change was not made in the University of Cambridge until John Haviland was Regius Professor of Physic in the 1840s, that is almost twenty years later.

Graves became one of the first physicians with a knowledge of anatomy

In these days a thorough knowledge of anatomy is an absolute requirement in the curriculum of medical schools the world over, but in the early nineteenth century the idea of a physician wishing to acquire such knowledge was unheard of. Thus it was that Sir William Wilde wrote in a biographical memoir of Graves after his death: "Having graduated in arts, Mr Graves applied himself to the study of anatomy, medicine and surgery, in the best schools of this city, and was among the first of the Dublin physicians who, following the path pursued by the celebrated Baillie were distinguished as accurate practical anatomists—for, previous to this period, the student of medicine (we mean of physic apart from surgery) required but a very limited knowledge of that most essential branch of his profession, and post-mortem examinations were never performed except by the surgeon. The result of this deficiency in medical education, and subsequent neglect in the practitioner, was that very little was then understood of that very important branch of science, the very basis of the healing art—pathological anatomy".

Finally in the year 1818 the young Graves graduated from Trinity with his MB or degree of Bachelor of Medicine, a qualification also recognised by the Royal College of Physicians, but he did not exercise this privilege officially until two years later when we see his name finally enrolled as a Licentiate of the College, LRCPI. This was the College of which he was soon to be elected a Fellow and in due course to serve as President from 1834 to 1835.

Chapter 6

Graves in Europe
The Men Who Shaped His Career

Graves who was now a qualified doctor was just twenty-two years old and he had already shown himself to be intellectually head and shoulders above his fellows, first at university and then at medical school. He was a striking young man with a swarthy, almost olive skinned complexion, black hair and penetrating eyes. A fluent speaker, he was the sort of person who commands attention in any company. It could fairly be said that he had the world at his feet, but what he now yearned for was a challenge.

In the last three years, as he followed the doctors on teaching rounds of their patients in Sir Patrick Dun's Hospital he had often been disappointed by the didactic teaching they provided with little science to support it. The spirit of Galen still lingered on with his ready answer for every problem in terms of a pragmatic medical philosophy, and treatment was usually by means of a multiplicity of herbal preparations, many of the constituents having no proven therapeutic value. Graves wanted to tackle diseases scientifically and his time with Perceval, the Professor of Chemistry, had not only laid the groundwork for such an approach, but Perceval had visited university centres in Europe and brought back ideas which fired in Graves a wish to travel and see for himself if the medicine being practised overseas was indeed superior to what he had experienced in Dublin. The upshot of all this was that he took what proved to be a momentous decision and planned a lengthy trip to embrace all the best centres he knew of in Europe. For the next three years he was to sit at the feet of the great men of medicine in England, Germany, Denmark and Scotland and it was their approach to medicine which moulded his subsequent thinking about diseases, about their treatment and, above all, the technique of imparting this knowledge to medical students. We really have to study these nineteenth century leaders of the new style of medicine in Europe and the methods by which they worked and taught, if we are to understand the complex character of the astonishingly mature doctor who returned to his native city of Dublin some three years later.

Meanwhile, the majority of his contemporaries went straight into clinical practice, for which they were inadequately prepared, learning often by their mistakes and picking up the necessary practical knowledge as best they could. Treatment at that time was largely empirical and there were few specific remedies apart from opiates for pain, mercury for syphilis which was administered by rubbing it into the skin as an ointment, and quinine for malaria. For the rest there were many preparations to be had from apothecaries' shops, but only a few of these, mostly derived from plants, have survived to the present day. Probably the best example is digitalis prepared from the leaves of the foxglove which was used as a diuretic to get rid of fluid, especially when the ankles swelled as they do in heart failure. It is still in use today as dried and powdered leaf or, more commonly, its active principle, digoxin, is prescribed. Prescriptions were always written in Latin, were elaborate and often contained many items of doubtful value merely included because they always had been. Polypharmacy, as the practice is now dubbed, was the order of the day and the finished product had to be attractively presented to the patient; 'elegant' was the word often used to describe it and the expression 'an elegant pharmaceutical preparation' still occasionally creeps into the advertising material of our modern drug houses.

Graves, had he been embarking on a medical career today in the British Isles would have sought medical posts first, as house physician, then as registrar and finally as senior registrar; appointments which can span a period of ten years or more in both teaching and district hospitals with the added hurdles of examinations which are set by the Royal Colleges. Such appointments simply did not exist in Graves' day apart from the rare senior medical apprenticeship. The élite of Dublin's students were wont to go to Edinburgh for a spell, mostly observing the senior physicians in their hospital practice or occasionally acting as unpaid assistants to their chief when he visited his fee-paying patients in their own homes.

Graves' quest for knowledge takes him to London

It is not difficult to imagine the excitement in the Graves' household when he announced his intention of going abroad, and the flurry of activity as his trunk was packed with, no doubt, loving care by his three young sisters. He was clearly aware that the clinical training of the embryo doctor in Dublin was woefully inadequate and reading between the lines of the various accounts of his professional life in memorials, obituary notices and the like, it is apparent that he was already toying with the concept of creating a new clinical medical school in his native city. Perhaps this best explains why when he arrived at his first stop, which was London, he presented himself to Sir William Blizard who had recently founded a new medical school attached to the London Hospital at Whitechapel in London's east end which was then, as it still is today, a deprived area with poverty and overcrowding. Its full title was the London Hospital Medical College and it is still one of the major teaching hospitals in the metropolis.

Sir William Blizard was a remarkable man, he was an auctioneer's son who had received very little schooling, but in due course was apprenticed to a surgeon in Mortlake, then a village on the banks of the Thames to the west of London, and it is known that he attended the great Sir Percival Potts' lectures at St Bartholomew's Hospital. He went to work as a surgeon at the London Hospital and was so highly regarded by his seniors that in the year 1780 he was appointed to the staff. Five years later in 1785 he founded the medical college with the help of a colleague, Dr Maclaurin, with whom he had for some time been running a private medical school similar to the coaching classes which still exist in London today. The actual founding ceremony was celebrated with an ode, for Sir William always celebrated every important event in his life by writing some verse about it. He was a meticulous person in both dress and habit who paid great attention to detail, was precise and clear in his diction and loved ceremonial of any kind. It was reported by the distinguished curator of anatomy at the Royal College of Surgeons, Sir Richard Owen, that the contrast between the shabby appearance of the public executioner, who was a surly fellow from Newgate prison and Sir William in immaculate formal clothes, added a bizarre and ludicrous touch to the sordid business of handing over bodies for dissection which, according to the law, had to take place in public in Cock's Lane. Graves was naturally attracted to the clinics and teaching of such an outstanding character as Blizard. Although the latter had had very little formal schooling he was intellectually outstanding and was made a Fellow of the Royal Society at the early age of forty-five. He was elected President of the Royal College of Surgeons on no less than two occasions and he received his knighthood in recognition of his contributions to medicine.

Graves had decided in his own mind and at an early age that a thorough grounding in the basic sciences was essential for a proper understanding of clinical science, a fact which has been lost sight of from time to time in the history of the Royal Colleges who are the arbiters of medical training and patient care in the British Isles. He had spent much of his time in the dissecting rooms of Dublin and had a first class grounding in anatomy which was then only considered necessary for those training to be surgeons, although even at this early stage there was little doubt that Graves was destined to become a physician. In addition he had already demonstrated a natural flair for physiology and chemistry, qualities which endeared him to Blizard.

The letters of introduction which Graves carried to friends of his own family living in London ensured that he tasted some of the social pleasures of metropolitan life; family ties between the two capitals have always been close. When he visited the Royal Colleges of both the physicians and the surgeons he was well prepared to enjoy their fine libraries and collections of portraits since those institutions so closely resemble in many particulars their sister Royal Colleges in Dublin. Graves was always a very competent artist in his own right and must have revelled in his visits to the art galleries of London which had the added attraction of being free. What a pity we are unable to trace any of the letters which he wrote home at this time. At this stage of his career the young Graves was in much the same category as the latter-day Rockefeller Travelling Fellow or Commonwealth Foundation Scholar from Britain who works abroad for a year or more on a plan broadly approved by his sponsors. The work undertaken is usually in part dictated by what his hosts can offer, but is also based on his own ideas and the outcome depends primarily on his own initiative. He had made enquiries and found out all he could about the leading centres of medical education and research in Europe before he left Dublin and then took the opportunity afforded by his stay in London to make further enquiries. As a result he chose well.

A look at clinical teaching in Germany
During the period of his travels while Graves was absent from his native Dublin from 1818 to 1820, Germany more than any other country in Europe had become esteemed for its medical schools and in particular their methods of clinical instruction. It was in this field that Graves particularly wished to see how the instruction which he had received at the bedside in Dublin might be improved. He now set out to see for himself in what way the Germans had advanced in clinical teaching, but at the same time he could never resist the attraction of following up any scientific advances which might in some way impinge on the medical scene. From both points of view his first choice of Göttingen could not have been bettered.

Göttingen University stands in the fine old Hanoverian city of that name which has strong historical links with England since it provided us with a royal family. It still has its mediaeval city hall and narrow winding cobbled streets and in the fourteenth century was an influential member of the Hanseatic League, that proudly successful cooperative of Baltic ports and cities which dominated the commercial scene for centuries. Subsequently Göttingen lost its important role, following the Thirty Years War, but then in 1734 George II founded the university. High academic standards were set and soon the city was one of the leading centres of learning in Europe and a Mecca for students. As with all universities there has to be some conflict between Town and Gown and in the case of Göttingen there was Die Göttingen Siebe -—the Göttingen Seven— when seven professors were expelled because they protested so vehemently at the withdrawal of their liberal constitution by the then King of Hanover.

When Graves arrived, the medical school was dominated by Professor Stromeyer (1776–1835) whose reputation was based on the fact that he was a first class theoretical chemist and amongst his other posts held that of General Inspector of Apothecaries Shops. This was comparable with the position held by Perceval in Ireland as Inspector of Apothecaries and this link provides the clue to Graves' choice of Göttingen. Today Stromeyer would probably be called a clinical pharmacologist and he had at this time an international reputation in what was still described as Materia Medica and Therapeutics as recently as fifty years ago. Clearly Graves enjoyed going the rounds with him in the hospital and attending his lectures. Indeed it was the standard of teaching at the bedside which most impressed him and which he immediately realised would have been so valuable to him when he had been a medical student back in Dublin. At last he was seeing the marriage of science and clinical practice in the treatment of patients at the bedside, the very basis of modern medical teaching.

The perpetual student
The other attraction for him in Göttingen was the presence of the renowned Professor Johann Blumenbach (1752–1840) who was something of a legend even in his own day. Blumenbach had been born in Gotha and educated in Jena and was currently holding the title of Professor of Medicine in Göttingen, but he was better known as a physiologist and above all as an anthropologist, a subject of which he is credited with being the father. At that time his reputation was based on the authorship of two particularly well known books: *Institutions Physiologicae* (1787) and more importantly his *Handbuch der Vergleichenden Anatomie* (1804) which we would translate as comparative anatomy. He was the leading pioneer in this subject, collecting skulls from every part of the world and devising methods of measuring them, and this at a time when explorers were opening up many new corners of the globe. He was not a great traveller himself and so had to depend on the writings of others for details of physiognomy, skin pigmentation, shape of nose, texture and coil of hair and much else besides. His old pupils sent him skulls and other material, but he was denied all the scientific aids upon which the modern geneticist relies: studies of haemoglobin types, the presence or absence of such enzymes as glucose-6-dehydrogenase and all the other tools of the trade. Despite all this he pioneered the classification of the human race into five great families—the Caucasian or white, the Mongolian or yellow, the Malayan or brown, the Negro or black and the American or red. It is easy to smile at this rather crude simplification today, but it really was the foundation of anthropology, a science which has latterly contributed much to the understanding of the biologist, the physician and in particular the haematologist.

It is particularly interesting for a present day doctor to see that the term Caucasian was first introduced by Blumenbach because it is still used to this day in American writing as a euphemism for someone of white European descent, indeed in recent years its use has been creeping into British medical publications and this at a time when it should be understood how inappropriate a term it is. Dr Bernard Freedman has recently drawn attention to the rather flimsy evidence on which Blumenbach based his choice of the word Caucasian. Freedman quotes Bendysh's wonderfully stilted English translation of Blumenbach's major work: *The Anthropological Treatises of Johann Friedrich Blumenbach* published by Longmans in 1865. Here is the relevant paragraph: "I have taken the name of this variety from Mount Caucasus, both because its neighbourhood, and especially its southern slope, produces the most beautiful race of men, I mean the Georgian; and because all physiological reasons converge to this, that in that region, if anywhere, it seems we ought with the greatest possibility to place the autochthons* of mankind. For in the first place, that stock displays,as we have seen, the most beautiful form of skull, from which, as from a mean and primeval type, the others diverge by most easy gradations on both sides of the two most ultimate extremes (that is, on the one side the Mongolian, on the other the Ethiopian). Besides, it is the white in colour, which we may fairly assume to have been the primitive colour of mankind. . . ."

It is not difficult to imagine how the young Graves, despite his deeply held religious convictions, revelled in the discussions which such original hypotheses provoked: sitting up long into the night arguing about these early concepts of evolution with his fellow students. It was not until 1835 that Charles Darwin visited the Galapagos Islands in HMS Beagle and it was a further quarter century before he published his great work *On the Origin of Species by Means of Natural Selection,* six years after Graves died.

Graves as his later professional life demonstrates so well was the perpetual student and during his travels he obtained a really liberal education. Not for him, to use his own words, "the life of a practitioner without practice" for he made himself intimate with the recent discoveries and modes of thinking in every school of medicine which he visited . Even at this stage he was forming friendships with the leading physiologists and physicians of Europe and he kept up a correspondence with many of them for the rest of his life. In all of this he was greatly helped by his extraordinary facility in acquiring foreign languages. Stokes recalls how on one occasion Graves went on a walking holiday in Austria and, having neglected to carry his

---

* Autochthon: Original, earliest known inhabitants, aborigines. OED.

passport with him, was arrested as a spy. What is more he was put into prison and when he protested that he was a British subject the authorities refused to believe him, for they asserted no Englishman could speak German as well as he could. He spent ten days in prison, Stokes tells us, before his identity was established and he was released.

Berlin introduces Graves to the study of infectious diseases
The next city in which he took up residence was Berlin and the interests which were kindled there were to last the rest of his life. As in Göttingen there were in Berlin at that time two outstanding men who clearly attracted him, Hufeland and Behrend, and their contributions to the medical school were largely complementary. Hufeland (1762–1840) was already at that time a very senior professor with all the respect and deference which that commands in a German university even to this day. Hufeland's reputation was based primarily on his contributions to the study of infectious diseases and he was the accepted authority on two of the worst scourges of his time, typhus and cholera. He was a prodigious author as the huge list of his publications demonstrates and Graves was to retain for the rest of his life a special interest in contagion and the spread of infection, both in his native country and on a global basis; no less than fourteen chapters of Graves' two volume *System of Medicine* are devoted to fevers and their treatment. Hufeland was also respected as a practical therapist and teacher of medicine and it was to him more than any other single person that Graves owed his excellent grounding in the treatment of infectious diseases which made up a great part of the work of a physician in his day. Hufeland had studied the spread of these diseases, not only locally but on a worldwide scale and he had formulated his own theory of contagion. Considering how little was known at that time about the causes of these conditions, his views were remarkably advanced for it has to be remembered that bacteria were not discovered for another thirty years. Graves, later in life, was to recount in his lectures how cholera had spread around half the world; indeed he predicted with considerable accuracy when it was likely to arrive in Ireland, where it did indeed arrive in 1831. Surely the germ of this idea must have been implanted in his mind by Hufeland.

The other shining light in Berlin at that time was Behrend (1803–1889) who was later to be recognised as the world authority on syphilis. Like tuberculosis, syphilis was in those days a great scourge there being no definite treatment for it such as we have today in penicillin. Thus a great deal of a physician's time was taken up in treating such patients, a course of treatment lasting many months or years. The introduction of the sulphonamides, next penicillin and finally the newer antibiotics has completely revolutionised the treatment of almost all the infectious diseases.

Management skills acquired in Denmark

Apart from his exploratory and often sightseeing trips to other countries, particularly France and Italy, of which more anon, he also studied with Professor Cohlston in Copenhagen. Professor Colsmann, as his name is spelt in Danish, was very much a product of the university, its hospital and in particular the department of surgery. Born in Copenhagen in 1771 he entered the university in 1788 attaining his surgical degree at the academy in 1797. He was appointed an assistant surgeon at the Royal Fredrik Hospital for a year and then did what must have appealed to Graves, he went abroad and studied for six years, most of the time in Paris. On his return home he took up once more his hospital appointment, married his professor's daughter and soon obtained the post of surgeon to the Royal Court. As Director General of Surgery in Denmark he must have been able to impart to Graves much wisdom on the administrative structure and management of medical services both within a university framework and within that of government.

This then in brief is how Graves spent his three memorable years abroad and as his later career progresses it is easy to see how the training he received moulded the pattern which it was to follow. His special interests were the logical outcome of his studies in Göttingen and Berlin and he did in due course found a new medical school just as Blizard in London had shown him how it could be done. But not all his time was spent in learning the new medicine, he was a man of wide interest and insatiable curiosity and so we must now follow him to France and Italy.

Chapter 7

Travellers' Tales
Graves Making the Grand Tour

Soon after Graves had settled down to work in Göttingen it is not surprising to find him making plans to travel to other centres in Europe and see for himself some of the famous places he had long heard about, the different people, the works of art and all those things which have attracted foreign travellers over the ages. It was comparable with the grand tour which the young man used to make in the eighteenth century in order to complete his education. Graves had such an enquiring and ingenious mind and in any case needed some relaxation from his medical studies. He used to write letters home to Dublin giving an account of what he had seen to Professor Perceval and an old fellow student called Russell who had been ordained priest: strict injunctions demanded that the letters were to be circulated around his friends. Unfortunately the letters themselves have not surfaced, but a rich source of quotations from them is to be found in William Stokes's introduction to *Studies in Physiology and Medicine by Doctor Graves,* a volume published as a memorial to him ten years after his death. The production of this book was clearly a work of love and the inscription on the fly-leaf reads:

This Volume, A Memorial of Graves, is, by his brother and by the editor, dedicated to Professor Trousseau. The brother referred to here is his elder brother, the Revd Richard Hastings Graves and of course the editor was William Stokes who had been in turn his pupil, assistant and colleague and now, ten years later, was Regius Professor of Physic in the University of Dublin.

The introduction which takes up the first eighty-three pages is a splendid memorial to Graves' life and work and contains not only excerpts from the original letters, but many interesting anecdotes; here is the first of them which tells how Graves met the great painter Joseph William Mallord Turner; it is so remarkable that it would be difficult to invent it.

Turner becomes Graves' companion
"During his sojourn in Italy, he became acquainted with Turner, the celebrated landscape painter, and was his companion on several journeys. He often spoke of the pleasure he enjoyed, during sketching tours taken in company with the great painter, the history of his first meeting with Turner may here be related: "Graves was

travelling by diligence, when, in one of the post stations on the Northern side of the Alps, a person took a seat beside him, whose appearance was that of the mate of a trading vessel. At first, no conversation took place between them, but Graves' curiosity was soon awakened by seeing his fellow-traveller take from his pocket a notebook, across the pages of which his hand, from time to time, passed with the rapidity of lightning. Overcome at length by curiosity, and under the impression that his companion was perhaps insane, Graves watched him more attentively, and discovered that his untiring hand had been noting down the forms of the clouds which crossed the sky as they drove along, and concluded that the stranger was no common man. Shortly afterwards the travellers entered into conversation and the acquaintance thus formed soon became more intimate. They journeyed together, remaining for some time in Florence, and then proceeding to Rome. Graves was himself possessed of no mean artistic powers, and his sketches from nature are full of vigour and truth. He was one of the few men in whose company Turner was known to have worked. The writer has heard him describe how, having fixed on a point of view, he and his companion sat down, side by side to their work. I used to work away he said, for an hour or more, and put down as well as I could every object in the scene before me, copying form and colour, perhaps as faithfully as was possible in the time. When our work was done, and we compared drawings, the difference was strange; I assure you there was not a single stroke in Turner's drawing that I could see like nature; not a line nor an object, and yet my work was worthless in comparison with his. The whole glory of the scene was there. The tone and fire with which Graves uttered these last few words, spoke volumes for his sympathy with, and his admiration of the great painter of nature."

"At times, however, when they had fixed upon a point of view, to which they returned day after day, Turner would often content himself on the first day with making one careful outline of the scene. And then, while Graves worked on, Turner would remain apparently doing nothing, till at some particular moment, perhaps on the third day, he would exclaim 'There it is' and seizing his colours, work rapidly until he had noted the peculiar effect he wished to retain in his memory. It is a curious fact, that these two remarkable men lived and travelled together for months, without either of them inquiring the name of his comrade, and it was not till they reached Rome, that Graves learned that his companion was the great artist".

All the evidence points to this extraordinary story being true and Turner was certainly a most unusual artist. He was born on April 23, 1775 at his father's barber-shop at 26 Maiden Lane near to Rules restaurant in Covent Garden, London. His mother went insane and his father taught young Turner to read but he had little else in the way of schooling, although by the age of nine he was already drawing and selling his work to help support the family. All his life he found it difficult to communicate by the spoken work. From an early age he liked to associate his work with people and places of historical and legendary interest and such was his skill with charcoal, water colours and oil that by the time he was twenty-eight, that is in 1803, he was elected a full member of the Royal Academy, had his own house off Harley Street and could begin to indulge his taste for travel. When he died in 1851, still something of a recluse, he left his money to provide a home for distressed artists and all the pictures in his studio, many of which he considered too good to sell to the public, to the nation, on condition that they housed them in their own gallery. It is only in 1987, 112 years later that his request has been fulfilled with the erection of the Clore Gallery next to the Tate on the Embankment. His notebooks, which are now in the study centre at the Clore Gallery, reveal that in 1819 he set out from London on August 1st and his route was Dover, Calais, Paris, Lyons, Grenoble and the Mount Cenis Pass, where Graves first met him. After visiting Turin, Como and Milan he explored the Simplon Pass, then to Verona, Venice, Bologna, Rimini, Ancona, Macerati and Foligno, arriving in Rome on 27th October. After only a few days he headed south to Naples where Graves also went and then he took in Herculaneum, Pompeii, where Graves was kept awake by Vesuvius, and then Amalfi, Sorrento, Salerno, and Paestum. The stamina of those travellers in the 1820s must have been phenomenal, especially when one considers the hazards they faced. Most journeys were made by coach including crossing the Alps. Eoin O'Brien in his life of Corrigan reproduces Turner's dramatic painting of Mount Cenis Pass which hangs in the Walker Gallery in Liverpool. The incident which this picture portrays of a coach capsizing in a snowstorm actually happened to Turner and he thoroughly enjoyed the excitement and sketching the scene, but this took place when he was on his return trip to England and not when he was accompanied by Graves. The rapid drawings which Graves comments on are to be seen in Turner's notebooks in the Study Centre.

Graves' letters home

Stokes also gives us quotations from more of his letters and they show Graves' great love of Latin tags and classical allusions at this time. Perhaps they were meant to impress his readers, many of whom had so recently been his teachers. This letter is headed Naples, December 21st, 1819:

"When Napoleon thought fit to imprison the present Pope, whose dominions then lay open to every invader, and from whose influence he could have had little to dread, the following from the book of Job, was written upon the door of the house in which the general sent to take the Pope prisoner, lived: '*Contra folium quod vento rapitur, ostendis potentiam tuam*'. When in Rome the Pope has been termed '*folium quod vento rapitur*'; may we not conclude that the temporal power of Rome is again dead; indeed, at present the kings of the earth seem as little influenced by the authority of the representative of St Peter, as by that of the remnant of the Roman Senate, for there still resides in the capital one senator. When the Papal Authority had made Rome a second time mistress of the world, when the bulls of the Christian Pontifex Maximus bore a sway as extensive as formerly did the edicts of her pagan imperial Pontifex Maximus, Rome's aspiring genius rising from amidst the tombs of her ancient heroes, seemed to console herself for the loss of her former power; but her consolation has now passed, and she stalks, the shadow of a shade, between the Vatican and the palace of the Caesars, mourning over the ruins of universal empire, twice gained, now lost for ever, I say for ever, because the character of its inhabitants, particularly the higher orders, is now so degraded, that there seems to be little chance of Italy's recovering her rank among nations".

Later he writes in lighter mood of those tormentors of travellers, bedbugs and fleas: "I shall now mention some of the miseries of Rome, which have continued to exist from Juvenal's time to the present, and in spite of their classicality, still annoy strangers. One of the great grievances common to ancient and modern Rome is the difficulty of finding any private house, much less any inn, where one can slumber undisturbed. Hence it came to pass that formerly many sick people died from want of sleep, and that it required great wealth to obtain a bedroom in the city free from the cause of disturbance, noise. But although nocturnal noises are no longer annoying in Rome, yet another cause of vigilance has succeeded still more general in its effects; for now not only the sick but the healthy are affected. Nor can wealth purchase exemption from its operations. This you will readily allow, Sir, when I tell you what I allude to is a certain animal which, together with 'culices' and 'rana palustres' may have robbed Horace of a night's rest on his journey to Brundusium. An English lady of noble birth was in so much dread of these creatures that she brought with her into Italy a portable iron bedstead, the feet of which she placed at night in a tub of water. Vain effort! Her ladyship had scarce passed the Alps before she bore visible marks of the inutility of this contrivance—*quis talia fando temporet a lachrymis*. A friend of mine was so tormented by their bites that when visiting the Capitol he flung, in a fit of rage, thirty of the ringleaders headlong down the Tarpeian rock!". Graves loved these classical allusions, thus from Naples December 3rd, 1819 he writes:

Last night I was awakened by the thunders of Mount Vesuvius, and am told that a smoking chasm has this morning been observed in the side of the mountain; the people seem to expect an eruption. If anything of this *vultus preclaera minantia* takes place, I shall let you know of it. I remember Sir, that when I was in Germany I formed a plan of describing that country to you as far as my observations and reading allowed me to do, but the wish to assist my observations by reading was the very cause of my abandoning that plan, for finding Madame de Stael's so complete as nearly to have exhausted all the most interesting subjects, and feeling that any attempt of mine to treat of the same subjects, would be like my endeavouring to retouch Raphael's pictures, I retired like Ariosto's Rodomonte vanquished by the enchanted spear of a female, and vowed not to use my arms, for a year, a month, a day; but my muse (an acquisition I have made by quaffing all sorts of poetical wines, from the Rhoetian to the Falernian) quoting the example of Lord Byron to prove that such vows are not now so scrupulously observed as they were by the knights of old, I break my vow with less remorse, and shall without adding to my already unreasonably long proemium, proceed forthwith to my peroratio."

Signs of home sickness
Writing to Russell, Archdeacon of Clogher, who was a great friend who had also been close to his brother Hercules, he sounds as if he is suffering from home sickness: "Although I have no doubt that you will be surprised, yet I am not without hopes that you will be pleased at receiving a letter from your quondam messmate and chess rival: if not I beseech you to bear your misfortune with patience, as the only amusement I have in my leisure hours is to sit down, and endeavour, as far as possible, to enjoy the idea, that by means of what I write I may, in some measure, carry on a sort of conversation with my friends. Here in solitude, and as it were in another world, where I am without connections, without friends, and stand completely insulated, I feel no small comfort in endeavouring to prevent those whom I value from forgetting me. When one is absent for any length of time from home, one soon forgets the common run of saluting acquaintances, and at the same time learns to set a proper value on those who are worthy to be called friends."

And later, again to Russell, from Aix en Provence, January 16th 1820: "I arrived here this morning from Marseilles, where I had spent the greater part of the night witnessing the follies of the last night of the Carnival, when I witnessed scenes in public which you could scarcely believe could have taken place; but I feel little inclined at present to give any account of them, as I have since paid a visit to what is to me the dearest spot in France, *viz* that which contains the remains of our beloved Hercules. Melancholy as it was,

I thank God that I have been able to perform it, as it is a scene that I can never remember without improvement. Immediately on my arrival here I was directed to the churchyard, which is on the outside of the wall of the town. After waiting some time, an old woman opened the door which leads into it, and I entered the abode of death with a strong impression of awe. It is about half an acre in extent, bounded on one side by the ancient wall of the city, and of a triangular shape. There are two doors, each with a cross on the wall above it. The greater part is devoted to the interment of Catholics, but there are but few tombs or graves in it. A wall three feet high divides the upper part, or Protestant burying ground. In the sketch I have marked with crosses a small chapel, and by H the grave of Hercules. The two other crosses mark the graves of an Englishman and a young English girl. The churchyard is very clean, decent, and well enclosed, which was to me gratifying. At the head of Hercules' grave there is a green marble stone with the following inscription: 'At Aix, on the 6th November, 1817, departed from this life, aged 22 years, Hercules Henry Graves, in the faith of Christ and the fear of the Lord.' This was, I believe, dictated by himself, and shows the judgement which formed one of the most valuable of his endowments, for he omits all the circumstances of his situation, country, etc, and only mentions about himself that he died in the faith of Christ and the fear of the Lord. 'Aged 22 years' made a deep impression on me. And am I then older than he? God forbid! Never did I so strongly feel how gratifying it must be to mark the spot of a departed friend with some token of remembrance; and had time permitted, I believe that I should have indulged myself with getting the names of his three friends inscribed on the tombstone."

Graves' actions when faced with dangers
This visit to the south of France with apparently no other purpose but to see his brother's grave in Aix, gives some idea of the extent of Graves' journeying in Europe. He was an inveterate traveller and when his letters have survived, an admirable reporter on both what he saw and what he heard. The traveller's tale which relates to this period and which never fails to receive a mention in any account of Graves' life is undoubtedly that of his encounter with a storm at sea in the Mediterranean. Anyone who has cruised in a sailing boat in that sea will have learnt to his cost of the suddeness with which foul weather blows up in that so-called inland sea and also the violence of the waves which have caused many a boat to founder. No doubt the story has lost nothing over the years with the retelling and, I suspect, the addition of "Merely corroborative detail intended to give artistic verisimilitude to an otherwise bald and unconvincing narrative" as W S Gilbert nicely expresses it. Here is William Stokes' account which I will quote verbatim:

"After leaving Rome he visited Sicily, and in connection with the excursion, the following incident is worthy of being recorded, as giving insight into his character, and as preparing us to estimate one of its features, for which in after life he was justly distinguished, namely, his promptness and vigour of action, when confronted with difficulty and danger."

"He had embarked at Genoa, in a brig bound for Sicily. The Captain and crew were Sicilians, and there were no passengers on board but himself and a poor Spaniard who became his companion and messmate. Soon after quitting the land, they encountered a terrific gale from the north-east, with which the ill-found, ill-manned, and badly commanded vessel, soon showed herself unable to contend. The sails were blown away or torn, the vessel was leaking, the pumps choked, and the crew in despair gave up the attempt to work the ship. At this juncture Graves was lying on a couch in the cabin, suffering under a painful malady, when his fellow passenger entered, and in terror, announced to him, that the crew were about to forsake the vessel; that they were then in the very act of getting out the boat, and that he had heard them say that the two passengers were to be left to their fate. Springing from his couch, Graves flung on his cloak, and, looking through the cabin, found a heavy axe lying on the floor. This he seized, and concealing it under his cloak, he gained the deck, and found that the captain and crew had very nearly succeeded in getting the boat free from its lashings. He addressed the captain, declaring his opinion, that the boat could not live in such a sea, and that the attempt to launch it was madness. He was answered by an execration, and told that it was a matter with which he had nothing to do, for that he and his companion should remain behind. "Then" exclaimed he, "it is a pity to part good company." As he spoke, he struck the sides of the boat with his axe, and destroyed it irreparably. The captain drew his dagger, and would have rushed upon him, but quailed before the cool, erect and armed man. Graves then virtually took command of the ship. He had the suckers of the pumps withdrawn, and furnished by cutting from his own boots the leather necessary to repair the valves. The crew returned to their duties, the leak was gained on, and the vessel saved."

This extraordinary tale, which is as imaginative as anything from Sinbad's Voyages must surely owe a little to the great skill of the Irish as raconteurs.

Chapter 8

The Traveller Returns
The Meath Hospital

The year 1820 saw the return of Graves to his native city of Dublin and wherever he turned, change was taking place. In London, George III, that typical Englishman, the Farmer King, with no English blood in his veins and few English words in his vocabulary, died, insane and blind. His son, the Prince Regent forsook his beloved Pavilion at Brighton and the charms of Mrs Fitzherbert to be crowned George IV in the following year. New buildings were going up in many parts of Dublin and one in particular was of especial interest to Graves. He had applied to the governors of the Meath Hospital for the post of consultant physician which had recently fallen vacant and in 1821 he was successful. For any young and ambitious doctor, his first appointment to the full staff of a hospital, and the Meath had in addition the prestige of being a teaching hospital, is the most important milestone in his career, and so it was with Graves who was eventually to become its most famous physician. The Meath, which was being rebuilt at the very time that he was appointed has had such a fascinating, if chequered history, that it is worth recalling here, especially as Graves was to play such a major role within its walls.

A time of social unrest
The very first Meath Hospital was opened on March 2nd 1753 for the care of the woollen weavers who at the time were suffering from severe unemployment and who lived in the surrounding district which was known as the Earl of Meath's Liberty. Much of Ireland's prosperity in the early years of the seventeenth century depended on the woollen industry and by 1698 some 12,000 Protestant families out of an estimated total Dublin population of 58,000 were employed in the trade. In 1700, envious eyes were cast on this prosperity by the English and as a result the Parliament in London passed an act prohibiting the import of woollens from Ireland. Thus it was that all the manufactured woollen goods made in Ireland were thrown on the home market which was only capable of absorbing a fraction of them. The outcome was that there were long spells of unemployment concentrated in the district, hunger was rife and it was not long before violence broke out.

Jonathan Swift, the Dean of St Patrick's Cathedral was the only man who could control the weavers and he acted as their leader. In

May 1734 a mob from the Liberty went into the city of Dublin to
seize the English manufactured woollens which were being allowed
entry into the country and were on sale in the shops. The drapers,
having been warned what was afoot, closed their premises securely,
but the infuriated weavers tore down the shutters and then proceeded to attack the sheriffs and bailiffs who turned out to try and
stop them. Eventually the army had to be called out and at least
eight people were killed or severely wounded. These riots continued
sporadically for some years; John Wesley in 1747 writes in his
journal of a visit to Dublin: "woe is me now, because my soul is
weary, because of murders which their city is full of! The Ormond
mob and the Liberty mob seldom meet, but one or more are killed.
A poor constable was the last, whom they beat and dragged about,
until they had killed him, then hung him up in triumph. None was
called in question for it; but blood covered the earth". Certainly
history confirms that violence has always been one of the essential
ingredients of life in Ireland as it is indeed, but happily to a lesser
extent, in most other countries.

From time to time most hospitals become unable to cope with the
heavy demands made on them, and in this respect the 1780s were
no different than the 1980s. Thus it was that the Governors of the
Meath Hospital started raising funds for a new building and public
subscriptions were set up. Each year a benefit play was held: in such
matters there has been little change over the centuries. There is a
record that in 1761 the manager of Smock Alley Playhouse, Thomas
Sheridan the father of Richard Brindsley Sheridan was invited to
perform, but then unfortunately, in 1770, a rather parsimonious
committee attempted to spare themselves the expense of such a
production and proposed having a charity sermon in St Patrick's,
this was quite rightly turned down. The alternative was a splendid
concert of Handel's works. The Irish have always been partial to
Handel since his Messiah had its world premiere in Dublin in 1742.

At last in 1773 the Governors had enough money to start building
a new Meath Hospital and this was done on a fresh site, the Coombe.
The hospital was then renamed the County of Dublin Infirmary.
With such a name it was guaranteed a steady income from the city
fathers, but within fifty years it was once again bursting at the
seams, this time because it had attracted such eminent staff. In
surgery it was particularly fortunate. Patrick Cusack Roney was
appointed surgeon in 1782 and following him both his sons served
the hospital well. The former was twice elected President of the
Royal College of Surgeons in Ireland. A little later William Dease
joined the staff, it was he who obtained the Royal Charter for the
Irish College of Surgeons and was their President in 1789; he is still
remembered as the author of books on midwifery and on head
wounds. A fine statue of him greets the visitor as he enters the hall

of the College of Surgeons on St Stephen's Green. Thus it was that yet again there was the necessity of rebuilding and the problem was to find a larger and more appropriate site.

The new Meath Hospital is built
Eventually an area covering about two acres with a wall all round it in Long Lane was considered ideal and purchased for £1,120, free of rent. This piece of land was none other than the garden or 'Long Walk' of Dean Jonathan Swift who had first leased it for his own use in 1725. At a later date he enclosed it with a fine wall nine feet high which cost the enormous sum for those days of £600. The wall was so that he could keep his horses there and because of the cost he called it Naboth's vineyard—it was not long before the locals called it 'Dean's Vineyard'. The architect for the new hospital, which was once more to be called the Meath, was William Farrell and it cost £11,716 to build.

Eventually the building was completed and it was decided to move in the patients from the old Coombe site on Christmas Eve 1822, Graves had only joined the staff one year before. It was a period of extremely foul weather and judging from contemporary newspaper reports this was not the only thing that was foul. During the days preceding Christmas the papers were full of protests against, and regrets for, the 'Orange Protest'. Thus the visit of the Marquess of Wellesley, Lord Lieutenant and elder brother of the Duke of Wellington, to a command performance of *She Stoops to Conquer* at the Hawkins Street theatre was marred by interruption from the one shilling gallery: "a quart bottle was thrown at the conductor who stopped the orchestra and held up the bottle; finally a watchman's rattle, a substantial piece of timber, ripped the cushion in front of His Excellency and rebounded between him and the chandelier of his box." Meanwhile, outside, the storm raged and while the patients, wrapped in blankets, were being carried from the Coombe in long baskets, slates dislodged by the gale fell about them. Indeed on the return journey the baskets were found very useful to protect the heads of the bearers. Many of the young surgeons actively assisted in this performance and two of the medical students who were happily returning to the old hospital holding baskets aloft were William Henry Porter who was to be president of the College of Surgeons in Ireland in 1838 and Maurice Collis who succeeded him as President in 1839.

Graves brings a new style of teaching to the new hospital
This then was the brand new hospital in which the recently appointed physician Graves was to initiate his innovative style of teaching medical students. We know precisely what he was setting out to do because he delivered an inaugural lecture at the medical

school giving his plans in detail and this speech is reported as the opening chapter of his major work *Lectures on Clinical Medicine*. Here are Graves' own words:

"The human mind is so constituted that in technical knowledge its improvement must be gradual. Some become masters of mathe-

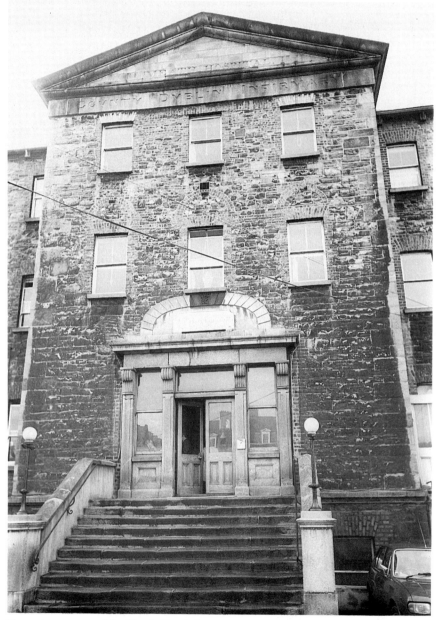

The main entrance of the Meath Hospital.

matics and of other abstract sciences with such facility, that in one year they outstrip those who have laboured during many. It is so, likewise, in the theoretical parts of medicine; but the very notion of practical knowledge implies observation of nature. Nature requires time for her operations; and he who wishes to observe their development will in vain endeavour to substitute genius or industry for time. Remember, therefore, that however else you may be occupied—whatever studies may claim the remainder of your time, a certain portion of each day should be devoted to attendance at a hospital, where the pupil has the advantage of receiving instruction from some experienced practitioner.

"A well arranged, and sufficiently extensive hospital contains everything that can be desired by the student; but, unfortunately, his improvement is seldom proportionate to the opportunities he enjoys. Whence this deficiency? How does it happen that many attend hospital day after day, year after year, without acquiring much practical knowledge? This may be attributed to want of ability or diligence on the part of the student, or to an injudicious or careless method of teaching on the part of the hospital physician. It may be well to examine in more detail the errors to which the students and the teacher are respectively most exposed". Then he goes on to list the various defects in medical education as he saw them at that time. First he points out that students should not aim at seeing many diseases every day but they should "constantly study a few patients with diligence and attention and anxiously cultivate the habit of making accurate observations". This cannot be done at once he says. The habit can gradually be acquired and he stresses that it is far more important to follow a few examples of disease in patients right through from start to finish than try and see a great many sick people.

He also argues against the student becoming too interested in the rarities encountered in medical practice and notes that many professors and authors are similarly affected with this bias, which may adversely affect their value as teachers. Then again he stresses the enormous importance of studying patients with chronic diseases for long periods, as opposed to those with acute conditions, which on the whole are more exciting to investigate and tend more readily to be treated successfully. He also complains of the overcrowding of the syllabus with too many subjects, and queries the value of spending long periods in the study of botany and pharmacology, chemistry and physics, when some of this time might be employed better in studying patients who are ill on the wards. His criticisms are as fresh and as relevant today as they were when he expressed them in Dublin more than 160 years ago.

Student education when Graves joined the staff at the Meath

He describes the current method of the day for teaching students. At that time the consultant would select from his senior pupils two clinical clerks, one to look after the male, the other the female patients. They would write up the patients' histories, make a careful examination and record the effect of the medicines given, noting any change in the symptoms since the physician's last visit to the ward. Then at his daily rounds the physician received the clinical clerk's notes and examined the patient whom he interrogated in a loud voice. This was necessary because all the students crowded round the bed, and with a big crowd in attendance those on the back rows could not hear. The patient's replies were repeated by the clerk in an equally loud voice. To use Graves' own words "to enable the whole audience to hear what is going on; but indeed, when the crowd of students is considerable, it is no easy task; it requires an exertion almost stentorian to render this conversation between the physician and his patient audible by the more distant members of the class; while the impossibility of seeing the patient obliged all who were not in his immediate vicinity to trust solely to their ears for information". Furthermore it was the custom at that time, and certainly so in Sir Patrick Dun's Hospital, to use Latin when speaking at clinics. Undoubtedly it was what we should refer to as dog Latin, and was still being used quite recently in the writing of prescriptions, so that the patient should not know what was in his medicine as written out by the physician.

Graves had other strictures on the methods then in practice, many of them stemming from his own sensitive and very humane approach to the sick. He thought it quite improper to mention serious diagnoses in the patient's presence and really unforgivable ever to suggest that there was little chance of recovery; he therefore adopted the method of taking the students to a nearby room where the individual clerk or dresser could be interrogated, the diagnosis and treatment freely discussed, and further management formulated. But his whole emphasis was on making the clerk feel that he was a member of a team treating the patient, that he was responsible for noting all that was going on and for planning the treatment, so that when he eventually qualified as a doctor he would be in a strong position not only to treat his own patients, but also to learn from their condition. Thus a practitioner's knowledge would improve as the years went by, something which unfortunately could not be said of many doctors at the time he was speaking.

We know from contemporary writings that Graves was a very courteous, kind and considerate doctor who would always sit at the bedside, not stand peering down on the patient as many doctors are still prone to do in hospital, and he took the time to listen and then discuss with the sick person the future problems which the complaint might produce. He was just as anxious that the student should behave likewise. He was constantly improving his own knowledge by reading, correspondence with other doctors, especially those he had met overseas, and by attending lectures and demonstrations, not only in the hospital wards, but in the pathology department.

Like all good doctors, Graves was the perpetual student. It is sometimes said today that postgraduate medical education starts on the day the medical student qualifies as a doctor and continues until he retires from practice. With the present day escalation in the pace of medical and especially therapeutic progress, this pattern of instruction has become a necessity if the practitioner is to keep abreast of new knowledge. Indeed in a lifetime of medical practice the average doctor will probably have to relearn a great part of what he mastered in his hospital years as a student, no matter which particular branch of medicine he has chosen to follow. The 1820s and 1830s were just such a time of wonderful medical and biological discovery.

Graves' changes were also occurring elsewhere in the UK

Maurice Collis who was a medical student at that time remarked that before Graves became their teacher, the number of clerks in the Meath Hospital used to average only ten, but after a very few years of Graves' teaching, the numbers had reached seventy. Over the ages students have always been good judges of their teachers. Another student of that time, Arthur Guinness, who qualified in 1835, writes of Graves that "He was a remarkably fine, tall man, dark complexion and hair. He was in my time the most hard working man of all the staff. He had a very large practice. He used to come in winter time, when I was a resident, about 7 o'clock in the morning when it was quite dark to visit the wards, and many a time I have walked round with the clinical clerk Hudson, and often carried a candle for Dr Graves." Many registrars and housemen of my own generation will recall similar episodes in their own apprentice days and for those unfamiliar with the routine of a teaching hospital, the 'working' rounds of the consultant staff are quite distinct from the more formal 'teaching' round which is held at a set time each week. Guinness goes on to say about Dr Graves, "and he told me on one occasion that, after he took his degree, he walked to Paris to visit the hospitals and from thence to Vienna walking the whole way to the latter city and returned home also on foot." There are few stories that do not improve with the years and with the telling and medical students are notorious for this. Despite this light hearted criticism it is abundantly clear that Graves left a remarkable and lasting impression on medical education in his own time which has lasted right down to the present day, replacing the old unsatisfactory 'walking the wards' and the lack of responsibility for care.

It would be wrong to believe that none of this new spirit of medical teaching had arrived in other parts of the British Isles and the equivalent of Graves in England was the physician John Forbes (1787–1861) who came from the West Country to practise at the Royal West Sussex Hospital in Chichester in 1822 and later moved to London where he eventually was appointed physician to Queen Victoria. He taught his students much as Graves did and was responsible for the first English translation of Laennec's Treatise on Diseases of the Chest published in Paris in 1821. It was in this book that the Frenchman, or should I rather say, Breton doctor, for he was a native of Quimper in Brittany, first described his new invention the stethoscope and placed the whole of chest diseases on a scientific basis. It is no coincidence that in 1825 William Stokes as a medical student in Edinburgh published a book on the stethoscope; it was Stokes who was to become Graves' favourite pupil, lifelong friend and colleague. The introduction of the stethoscope heralded a new and more scientific approach to the clinical diagnosis of diseases of the heart and lungs, which for centuries had been dominated by a kind of ceremonial or mystic laying on of hands and feeling of the pulse. Science was at last coming to the bedside and what we can now recognise as the 'Age of Measurement', which is still with us, was dawning.

Graves saw the student as a fellow worker

Graves was the first to raise the medical student from the position of an inferior, who was simply permitted to look on and trail along in the footsteps of a very grand man, often indeed hardly able to hear what was being said, and to elevate him to the position of a fellow worker with the visiting physician. What is more he insisted that the student join him daily, observing and recording the changing symptoms and signs in the sick patient and in addition he had to share the responsibility in the daily plan of treatment. This, combined with excellent clinical instruction meant that the student could eventually stand on his own two feet as a skilled and even scientific practitioner. Graves encourged questions and was always willing to discuss the points which he had raised; perhaps even more importantly he was both truthful and humble about the mistakes which he himself had made. He insisted on attending the post-mortem examinations on his own patients and others who died in the hospital, claiming that this was the only way to learn about disease and about the effects of treatment.

One hundred years later the great Sir William Osler, Canadian born, the foundation Professor of Medicine at Johns Hopkins University in Baltimore and finally Regius Professor of Medicine at Oxford, was to repeat the almost identical message and in practising his own precepts, always attended the post-mortem room and learned from his own and others' mistakes the correct diagnosis of disease in those patients who had been studied and treated, but succumbed in the wards. The lunch-time post-mortem demonstration in front of the consultant and resident staff with their students is still, today, the hallmark of those hospitals which command most respect for their standards of care and for their contributions to new knowledge in medicine. For even the most skilled consultant it can still be a very humbling experience.

The stethoscope arrives in Ireland

It was Graves who first introduced Laennec's stethoscope to Ireland and used it at the Meath Hospital. Andrew Young, who was a student working there at that time recollects how "there was much surprise and no little incredulity with a shade of opposition shown by sneering, or, as we now say, by 'chaffing', on its first introduction. The juniors looked at it with amazement as a thing to gain information by—it so put them in mind of the pop-gun of their schooldays; the seniors with incredulity. The first implement of the kind I saw was a piece of timber (elm I think) about the scantling of an ordinary modern beetle [wooden mallet] three inches diameter, 12–14 inches long, having a hole driven through it from top to bottom, all one piece and no attempt at any kind of ornamentation." Graves' enthusiasm for the stethoscope stemmed from the information his protégé Stokes brought him from Edinburgh where he qualified as a doctor in 1823. Stokes was enthusiastic about his new diagnostic tool and wrote a thesis on the subject for his degree. Graves as usual immediately tried one, realised its potential, and made himself proficient in its use.

A good idea of the impact of Graves' teaching was provided by Trousseau, the chief of medicine at the Hotel Dieu in Paris, in his introduction to the French translation of Graves' book *Clinical Medicine;* in a fulsome tribute he includes the following paragraphs which were rendered officially into English as follows:

"Graves is an erudite physician; while so rich in himself, he borrows perpetually from the works of his contemporaries, and at every page brings under tribute the labours of German and French physicians. Although a clinical observer, he loves the accessory sciences; we see him frequently having recourse to physiology, in the domain of which he loves to wander; to chemistry with which he is acquainted, which he estimates at its true value, and to which he accords a legitimate place.

"Graves is often empirical. What true clinical observer can avoid being so? But he is so in spite of himself. He seeks, he points out the reasons which determine him; he discusses them, and he conducts his pupil step by step from the theory, occasionally too ingenious, to the application, which is always useful, though often unexplained.

"Graves is in my acceptation of the term, a perfect clinical teacher. An attentive observer, a profound philosopher, an ingenious artist, an able therapeutist, he commends to our admiration the art whose domain he enlarges, and the practice which he renders more useful and fertile."

This official translation of Trousseau's foreword conveys the meaning while doing scant justice to the splendid French of the original.

Chapter 9

Graves as a Family Man

Graves never ceased surprising everyone with his immense drive and boundless energy. He returned from Europe in 1820 and had only been back in Dublin a few months when he opened his consulting rooms and having made a considerable impact on the medical profession, obtained an appointment to the staff of the Meath Hospital whose new buildings were nearing completion. Then in 1821 he married; it must have been a whirlwind romance, the bride was Matilda Jane, daughter of Richard Eustace, and in due course a little girl was born whom they christened Eliza Drewe Graves. Meanwhile, out in the west of the country they were suffering from one of the recurrent outbreaks of potato blight which in the first half of the nineteenth century struck Ireland, and to a lesser extent other countries in Western Europe, with such regularity. The result was starvation for many in Galway and there followed an epidemic of typhus as many of the poorest folk flooded into the city. The Lord Lieutenant from his headquarters in Dublin put out an appeal for doctors to go to the stricken area and Graves with his consuming interest in epidemics, infectious fevers and their spread, gathered a team of five young doctors around him and set off to Galway at once.

The people worst hit by famine were the peasants of Connemara and as they had nothing to eat they moved into the city of Galway. Their desperate poverty, which led to overcrowding and undernourishment, provided the ideal conditions for infestation with body lice in which the typhus organisms live as parasites. Typhus epidemics have been described ever since history was first recorded and it can be a fatal disease, so that the doctors who had volunteered to work among the sick were running a serious risk. The fever hospital in Galway could not cope with the vastly increased numbers so huts and tented wards were erected in the surrounding grounds. The doctor in charge of the hospital died of typhus and so did two of his successors, a tragedy which was to recur on an even greater scale among Irish doctors during the disastrous potato famine in 1845. It is not difficult to imagine the anxious state of the young Mrs Graves as the news travelled back to Dublin; how she must have missed the support of her husband. Graves gives us a graphic account of what it was like in the epidemic, in one of the first papers he ever wrote, in the *Transactions of the Association of the King and Queen's College of Physicians for 1824,* a publication which is now something of a rarity in medical libraries.

Graves widowed twice

Graves returned to Dublin and in 1823 was elected a Fellow of the Royal College of Physicians of Ireland, the highest diploma which they could confer on him. With his customary vigour he threw himself into even greater activity and with his medical colleagues founded a new medical school called the Park Street School of Medicine which was to survive for twenty years. He was certainly putting to good use his recently acquired knowledge from his European tour, first the teaching of Hufeland on fever epidemics in Berlin served him well in Galway and then Blizard's experiences in setting up a new medical school in London provided a blue print for Park Street. But 1825 brought tragedy to the Graves' home, little Eliza died and then in September, so did Graves' wife Matilda, and so before he was thirty years old he was already a widower.

Now Graves had been collaborating with Professor Brinkley who held the appointment of Astronomer Royal of Ireland as well as being Professor of Astronomy in Trinity. John Brinkley was born in 1763 in Suffolk and graduated from Caius College, Cambridge, as senior wrangler in mathematics. Although Brinkley was so much older than himself, Graves had found him a willing colleague in calculating the probability with which certain epidemics such as cholera spread, and had found him uncannily correct in predicting dates using the information which Graves culled from colleagues overseas. It is clear that Graves was always at his best when collaborating with older people rather than those of his own age. Another bond was that both men were devout Christians, indeed John Brinkley was later consecrated Bishop of Cloyne having been ordained priest many years previously while still lecturing on astronomy in the university. It is therefore not so surprising that almost exactly a year after his first wife Matilda died, that is in September 1826, Graves married Sarah Jane Brinkley, the daughter of his friend and colleague the Astronomer Royal. But tragedy was to strike again and although a daughter was born to the couple in 1827, whom they christened Sarah-Jane, note the hyphen, the mother died soon after and the child also succumbed. In these privileged days, more than 150 years on, when most of us enjoy excellent health care, it is easy to forget the devastating mortality which prevailed at that time, not only the neonatal and infant mortality, but adults also had a much reduced expectation of life. Graves once more busied or one might say buried himself in his work, his private practice became extensive, he instituted four o'clock lectures at Sir Patrick Dun's Hospital which was the hospital associated with Trinity, and his publications appeared almost monthly in the medical journals. These contributions to medical knowledge were so valuable that many of them were being re-printed shortly afterwards in the journals in London. Among the group of distinguished doctors who were then gracing the Dublin scene, Graves was undoubtedly *primus inter pares.*

Graves' third wife and her grand social ambitions

If we can now briefly set aside his professional career and concentrate on his social life, we find that four years later, in 1827, Graves was once again contemplating matrimony, but strangely on this occasion his choice fell on someone absolutely different in character and background from his first two wives. Anna Grogan was the daughter of the Revd William Grogan of Slaney Park, a fine house on the outskirts of the country town of Baltinglass which lies on the borders of Co. Kildare and Co. Wicklow. The Grogans are an old and distinguished Irish family who have occupied Slaney Park since the 1600s. Anna's parents were very much in the mould of what the English today call 'county' and Anna was brought up to be socially conscious and take a leading part in local events, which included the annual visit to Dublin, when the young ladies appeared in all their finery at dinners and dances to be partnered by eligible young men.

My wife and I drove our hired car down from Dublin due south to Baltinglass, it is only about thirty-five miles, to have a look at the Grogan's old family home. Not knowing how to find it we called in at a grocer's store on the town's main street and asked the way to Slaney Park. The immediate response was for the assistant to step outside the shop saying "Oh you want the Grogans' house up the hill there" and an arm shot out to indicate a rise less than a mile away. It was exciting to know that Grogans were still living there, the locals must have been directing people in just such terms for more than 300 years and, as usual, it is the name of the family and not what they call their house which identifies it in the neighbours' eyes. We did just as we were directed and drove up a hill from which an avenue led us up to a front door. A knock was greeted by much barking from a young Doberman Pincher backed up by some deep throated retrievers and soon the door opened and we were greeted by Mrs Grogan, an Englishwoman born and bred and soon after by her husband who had to come in from the farm. They told us how they had let their house to a local doctor while they were absent on war service and sadly it had been disastrously damaged by a fire so that most of the original contents had either been destroyed or looted. To compound the damage, the upper storey had never been replaced and what had once been a very lovely Queen Anne house now lacked all its old symmetry and charm. It then transpired that the architect who had been responsible for the 'restoration' had been none other than Manning-Robertson, the husband of Graves' grandaughter Nora Robertson the author of that charming book *Crowned Harp*, and the owner of Huntingdon Castle in Clonegal

where our researches had really first begun. We were disappointed
to find that there were no old pictures or mementoes of Anna Grogan
and the days when Graves had been courting her. However the
present day Grogans had heard about Graves and his marriage to
their ancestor.

Returning to 1830, Anna Graves as she now was, proved to be of
much more durable stuff than either of Graves' previous two wives,
she not only produced a family of six, two boys and four girls, but she
also outlived him for twenty years. The youngest girl was 'Little
Flo'. The picture of Anna which is conjured up for us by the
reminiscences of Little Flo's daughter, Nora Robertson, is of a tiny
good looking woman with a tough, even hard character, no intellectual interests, but excellent taste in artistic matters. Bright, hard
and probably brittle, she collected objets d'art with skill and some
are still treasured by her descendants, like the lovely huge famille
verte bowl which had been looted from the Imperial Palace in
Peking by an ancestor. When young she had been most active in the
social life around her home in Baltinglass and when she married
Graves and settled into the social life of Dublin she was soon well
known for her entertaining and her social success is certainly

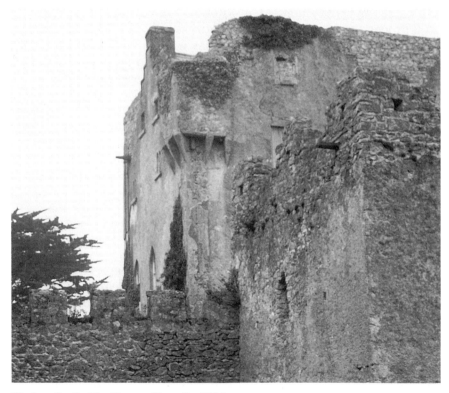

Cloghan Castle. The Norman Keep. Co. Offaly.

confirmed by her grand-daughter Nora Robertson who writes: "My mother, Florence, youngest child of Dr Robert Graves, FRS, was a born radical, how it came about I do not know. Her most conventional and decorous mother, Anna (nee Grogan of Slaney Park, Baltinglass), certainly never alluded to the family rebel, Cornelius, of Johnstown Castle, Co. Wexford, whose end was tactfully passed over in Burke as 'died in 1798', while his respectable ensign brother is recorded as 'fell' in the same year at the battle of Arklow. Coming from a county family, it was a constant irritant to my grandmother that her husband was a doctor. She worked the eminence to which he rose so adroitly that the Lord Lieutenant and his lady actually dined with them in Merrion Square. Still, she could not feel that this imprimatur was as enduring as founding a country seat and, before his death, she persuaded him to buy Cloghan Castle, a distinctive Norman Keep by the Shannon, near Banagher".

A prominent rôle to play in society

Anna was more than anxious that she and her husband should play a prominent rôle in the society of the day and Dublin was by all accounts a very attractive and gay city in the early 1800s. They moved into a large house on the south side of Merrion Square, Number 4 is I believe today Number 55, and to live at that time in such a house was the height of fashion. Graves' friend William Stokes lived at 5 Merrion Square North and Sir William Wilde eventually took the corner house, Number 1. I have been shown a charming little envelope of that period, edged in red and closed with sealing wax impressed with a coronet, containing a tiny sheet of notepaper headed Portobello Barracks, Thursday.

"Lord Mount Charles presents his compliments to Dr and Mrs Graves and has much pleasure in accepting their invitation for dinner for Friday [this is crossed out] Saturday June 6th."

The notepaper heading is beautifully embossed with his lordship's initials surmounted by an earl's coronet. The envelope is addressed to Mrs Graves at 4 Merrion Square S. No doubt Anna kept this little envelope as a memento of one of her successful dinner parties.

By 1827 Graves had been appointed Professor of the Institutes of Medicine as it was called at Trinity and he was visiting the Meath Hospital daily, as we have seen, often very early in the morning. On top of this he had a huge private practice which entailed spending much time in his consulting rooms and, in addition, many of the sick had to be visited in their own homes. Finally he had his lectures to prepare; every afternoon at four o'clock precisely, he was a very punctual person, he would deliver a lecture in the amphitheatre of Sir Patrick Dun's Hospital. Graves was a very very busy man and had little time for social occasions, it was this which irked his wife

Anna. However, he needed a substantial income to provide for the sort of expenses which his family were incurring, it was certainly a large family by modern standards consisting of two boys and four daughters.

The country seat is bought

Anna's next ambition, as her grand-daughter tells us, was indeed to have a country seat, but it was not until the early 1840s that she was able to persuade her husband to consider it, by then of course he was well enough off to purchase and maintain such an establishment. Graves' private practice had grown to the point where he had to limit the number of patients he saw in order to continue with his writing and research. He had also taken time off to visit clinics on the continent and such journeys by packet boat and horse carriage were very slow by today's standards. It is difficult to see how Graves would have had much time to visit, far less to live in his country home, although he did resign from his Chair of Medicine in 1841 and from the staff of the Meath Hospital in 1843. Eventually in 1852 Anna had her way, but Graves had little time left to him for he died of cancer of the liver in 1853.

It is interesting to see what happened to the Graves' children. The eldest boy Richard was born in 1832 and when his father died he was just twenty-one years old. Like his grandfather and his uncle

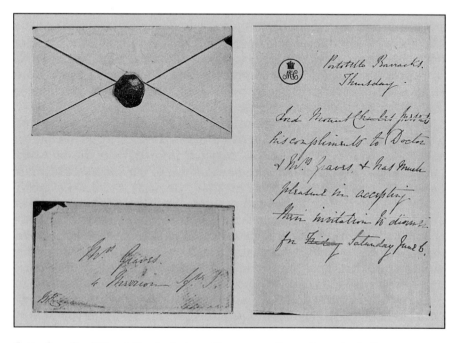

Letter from Lord Mount Charles to Anna Graves accepting a dinner invitation.

before him he was ordained priest and later he married Henrietta
Leathers of Herringfleet Hall in Suffolk. They had three children,
one daughter married into the Synge family, famous for the Irish
playright JM Synge, author of *Playboy of the Western World.*
Richard died in Milan in 1871 and his brother William, three years
his junior, who had by then become a colonel in the army, inherited
Cloghan Castle when his mother died in 1873. The Graves' four
daughters, Georgina, Elizabeth, Olivia and Little Flo were all married from the castle: Georgina in 1857 to a son of the Lord Chancel-
lor, how pleased her mother Anna must have been! Elizabeth to a
major in the army, Olivia to a KC with whom she moved to
Montreal, and finally Little Flo who married her major at the local
garrison in Birr who later had such a distinguished career.

Cloghan Castle looks the epitome of an old Norman Keep with a
fine residential wing which was added in 1820. The original castle
was built in 1120 in the reign of Henry I by Sir John MacCoughlan,
his wife Sabina O'Daly paying all the expenses. Both families bear
names famous in Irish history as do the O'Maddens the next
owners. In 1595 Queen Elizabeth I's representative, Sir William
Russell who was the Lord Deputy besieged the castle, set fire to the
thatched roof and then sacked it throwing six of the inmates over
the ramparts to their death.

It was in 1852 that Cloghan Castle came on the market and here
is the estate agent's advertisement for it:

Cloghan Castle Estate.

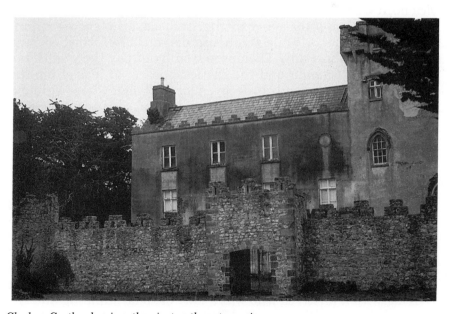

Cloghan Castle, showing the nineteenth century wing.

All well sheltered, fenced and walled, within two miles of the town of Banagher and half a mile of the banks of the Shannon. Built in the reign of King John, it is handsomely situated in the centre of the demesne and considering its great age is in a fine state of preservation. It is four storeys high, having three doors which open on the top, north, south and east. It contains three cellars, hall, pantry, drawing room, state bedroom, two other bedrooms, nursery and three servants' rooms attached to the Castle; on the south side is the kitchen, servants' hall and scullery together with a large store, loft or bedroom. There is a new addition on the east side, forming a comparatively modern building three storeys high, containing parlour, drawing room, three bedrooms and hall.

This must have been exactly what it was like when Anna moved in. We went to look at it in 1985, driving seventy miles due west of Dublin until we arrived at the little town of Banagher. Here it was that Anthony Trollope lived when he was the local postmaster and acquired his great love of the hunting field. Here too came Charlotte Bronte to marry the Revd Mr Bell and spend the rest of her life in the Old Rectory. When at last we discovered the castle, almost a mile up a disused drive, it was all shuttered and barred; the surroundings were neglected and overgrown but even this could not detract from its majestic and rather forbidding exterior. Indeed it looks precisely as it should; gaunt, massive, yet splendidly proportioned, because the Normans were great builders as their cathedrals throughout the British Isles and the continent so eloquently bear witness. In 1972 it was bought by Brian Thompson who was born in New Zealand to Irish emigrant parents. In 1976 he donated the surrounding 1500 acres to the Irish government as a bird sanctuary and for a while the house, beautifully furnished, was open to the public. Sadly Thompson would not pay the wealth tax and so left for Canada and the castle appears, at least from the outside, to be going rapidly to decay. A local villager whom we found tending the cows which were grazing what had once been the lawn said that anything of value had been stripped out and sold, including the old coach, a cannon from the battlements and even some of the doors. We found no way of getting permission to enter.

The pressures on Graves' family life

Now Cloghan castle is a good seventy miles from Dublin, the roads were not good in Graves' day and the journey by coach must have been a considerable undertaking in the 1840s. Thus Graves, completely immersed in his work and not much more than a year left to him, saw little of his wife Anna and the family. Indeed some members of the family have told us that in his later years he took to living with a mistress who was a lady of some standing and she bore him children. When he died from liver cancer he was only fifty-five and his wife paid for the extra-marital children's education for by that time husband and wife were reconciled. All this is hearsay evidence only. Unfortunately the correspondence relating to this period of his life was burned by a grand-daughter we were told. One of the great grandchildren remembers going into the library at Huntingdon Castle and surprising her in the act. She was anxious she said that there should be no blot on the family escutcheon!

The Graves' estrangement, although only a temporary one in their case, is often seen to this day in those échelons of the medical profession when a consultant physician or surgeon becomes greatly in demand. Not only are there calls on his time both by night and day in order to cope with patients suddenly taken ill, but there are so many other calls on him. There is the necessity to attend professional meetings, which are almost always in the evening, so that a wife hardly sees her husband except for those few hours, when exhausted by his overburdened schedule, he lays his head on the pillow and more often than not immediately falls asleep. He will also be expected to attend meetings in other cities, at home and abroad, and may well be called on to give papers and lectures, all of which means further time-consuming activity at his desk and in libraries. People much in the public eye are particularly susceptible to flattery and it is not so surprising that such men have fallen captive to the blandishments of younger women with whom they find themselves working, and as a result, finally separate from their wives.

It appears to me that in his late forties Graves developed a moderately severe mental depression and then turned against his wife for some years. He withdrew largely from public life except for his private practice, first resigning from his Chair of Medicine in 1841 when he was forty-five years old. He was persuaded to be President of the Royal College of Physicians of Ireland in the session 1843 to 1844 and then he abruptly resigned from his beloved Meath Hospital which he had served in an honorary capacity for twenty-three years. His colleagues were very upset by this move and sent a delegation to wait on him at his home and try to persuade him to remain, but to no avail. Whether or not he had a mistress during this difficult period is not clear but it seems more than likely. However he was eventually reconciled with Anna and this might well be the reason for Little Flo being so much younger than her brothers and sisters. Without solid evidence to support it this is pure supposition and it is true that many families do have a child late in married life, a child often referrred to as an afterthought.

Little Flo and Anna Graves remain at Cloghan Castle

After the death of her husband, Anna Graves remained in Cloghan Castle with Little Flo who was more than twelve years younger than any of her other children. Cloghan must have been a frightening place for a small child and very soon her brothers and sister, being so much older, left home and she had no one to play with. Here it was that her mother as the widow of a distinguished Dublin doctor and past President of the Royal College of Physicians brought her up and she subsequently met her husband, who was an officer in the nearby garrison town of Birr. He had a most distinguished career both at home and in India. Having raised the XVIth Irish Division in the 1914–1918 war, he was too old to take them to Europe. Finally as Lieutenant General Sir Lawrence Worthington Parsons he died at the age of 73. His younger brother was the inventor of the Parsons steam turbine and his elder brother was a Fellow of the Royal Society and an astronomer. Thus Little Flo married into a distinguished and very gifted family.

Lady Parsons' daughter Nora recalls vividly the stories her mother told her of being brought up as a little girl at Cloghan Castle. She writes:

"My mother's account of those days included; reading the classics in the worst light concealed under heavy furniture; of the sound of the maid's vanishing footsteps down the stone spiral steps from the attic bedroom when she was crying herself to sleep from fright; of the happy Sunday breakfasts when, instead of plain 'stirabout' [i.e. porridge] she was allowed the treat of the top of her mother's boiled egg. The rest was policmen; kind RIC constables were her playmates at birds' nesting and helping her to ride. Her mother was a harsh landlord and, therefore, under constant 'protection'. My mother, no doubt mindful of the egg-top, was fond of the hard, beautiful woman and hoped that she would not be shot; but even then felt that, if she were, she richly deserved it." That is the only account that we have of Graves' wife; perhaps the family gossip that they were estranged for some years and hence the long gap before 'Little Flo' was born, has some foundation in fact.

Nora Parsons, the grand-daughter of Graves married an architect, Manning Robertson; she records in her own handwriting in her book of the family tree:

Nora Kathleen Parsons born May 2 1887 Baptised All Saints, Norfolk Square, original church burnt. Godparents Revd and Honble, Randal Parsons, Mrs Seymour, Mrs Farmer.
m Oct 15 1912 at St Peters Eaton Square
Manning Durdin Robertson
in Burke's Landed Gentry; Robertson of Huntington Castle.

Chapter 10

Graves as His Contemporaries Saw Him

For almost twenty years, from the middle of the 1820s to the mid 1840s, Graves dominated the medical scene in Dublin. As the doyen of physicians, teaching, lecturing, writing and receiving foreign visiting doctors, he was the leader of the renaissance of medicine in Ireland and we are fortunate in having a couple of pen portraits of him, both written anonymously during his lifetime. One is by his boyhood friend and near neighbour William Wilde and the other by the *Lancet*'s correspondent, Erinensis. Finally to add a critical note there is the 'Gibson Affair', the remarks made by a physician from Philadelphia.

The contemporary writings of Erinensis
Let us take Erinensis first, this was the nom de plume of Dr Herris Green who was the talented, ribald and witty correspondent and medical critic acting as the *Lancet*'s man in Dublin in the days when Wakley, its founder editor was at his most rumbustious. Herris Green qualified as a doctor at Trinity a few years after Graves and went to London where he studied and obtained the membership of the Royal College of Surgeons. Returing home, he was for eighteen years the anonymous correspondent of the *Lancet*. He was brilliant at his task, could translate articles from French and German for the Journal and eventually returned to London to become Wakley's sub-editor. His latter days were spent in England where he joined the council of the British Medical Association, the BMA, and then in 1840 was co-editor with RJ Stratton at Worcester of the *Provincial Medical and Surgical Journal* which was the forerunner of the present day *British Medical Journal*. We know all this because of the researches of Martin Fallon who is a present-day surgeon recently practising in St Andrews and Dundee, and the author of a splendid biography of a contemporary of Graves, the surgeon Abraham Colles of Dublin, the bicentenary of whose birth was celebrated in 1973. It was this introduction to the subject which led Fallon in 1979 to edit a collection of the articles culled from old copies of the *Lancet;* they are witty, stylish devastating in their perceptiveness; they certainly would never see the light of day in modern medical journals.

Much of what was published in the medical press of those days would be grounds for a libel suit today, but the *Lancet* was so successful in stirring the medical pot that it was instrumental in

starting all manner of reforms. On November 8th 1828 there was a
long account from Erinensis describing the opening of the medical
session for the current academic year in Dublin. At that time there
were very many private medical schools in the city as well as those
of Trinity and the College of Surgeons. Erinensis must have visited
most of them and then proceeded to review their various perform-
ances in critical and often scathing terms, but always with touches
of humour. It is true that some of the schools were quite inadequate
in what they taught or expected from their pupils, but they must
have been profitable for their owners or there would not have been
so many of them; the excuse that was put forward was the urgent
need to train doctors to serve in the Armed Forces. Kirby's course
for those who wanted to join the army was typical of this sort of
'school', and was so successful that the certificates he issued were
even being forged in London. Here is how Erinensis described one
of Kirby's lectures, it is an excellent example of his reporting.

"For the purpose of demonstrating the destructive effect of
firearms on the human frame, Bully's Acre (a paupers' graveyard)
gave up its cleverest treasures for the performance of the experiment. The subjects being placed with military precision along the
wall, the lecturer entered with his pistol in his hand, and levelling
the mortiferous weapon at the enemy, magnanimously discharged
several rounds, each followed by bursts of applause. As soon as the
smoke and approbation subsided, then came the tug of war. The
wounded were examined, arteries were taken up, bullets were
extricated, bones were set, and every spectator fancied himself on
the field of battle, and looked on Mr Kirby as a prodigy of genius and
valour for shooting dead men".

At that time, bodies for dissection were both plentiful and inex-
pensive because of the activities of the Resurrectionists as the body
snatchers were called. Today, Mr Kirby's portrait looks down
benignly on the visitor as he mounts the main staircase of the Royal
College of Surgeons in Ireland overlooking St Stephen's Green.

Here then is the report of the opening of the academic year for
1828 at the School of Physic in Sir Patrick Dun's Hospital, which
was the clinical medical school of Trinity. The Professor of the
Practice of Medicine, whose name was Grattan, gave the inaugural
lecture and this is what Erinensis said about him:

"An extreme pallor of countenance marked by a sickly lividity
under the eyes, a broad and smooth forehead spanned at the base
by a pair of spectacles; a very weak and pharisaically modulated
voice with a general aspect of devotional abstraction, would stamp
him rather as an expounder of the Gospel than a commentator on
Celsus or Cullen. His lecture being on the hackneyed subject of
medical history, we of course exercised our peculiar prerogative of
criticising it asleep, and we can only say, that it had at least the

merit of evincing an acquaintance with the original authorities from which these encyclopaedic compilations are drawn, which furnish information to other lecturers, such as Mr Adams, at second hand. . . ."

Erinensis describes Graves

Then comes a pen portrait of Graves which in its exaggeration is the equivalent in words of a cartoon by Spy.

"Dr Grattan was succeeded, at a short interval, in the same theatre by the Professor of the Institutes of Medicine, a gentleman of a very different appearance and cast of mind. Had we not been aware that Dr Graves had the supreme honour of being born in Ireland, we would be inclined to set him down as a native of the south of Europe. His colour is a rich bronze or brown olive far too deep to be burned on by the coy sun of Ireland, which shrouds his glory too often in an unpenetrable veil of clouds to darken the fair complexions of his children. His hair is of that intense black and glossy texture, which is found to perfection in warmer latitudes only; while his keen black eye, sparkling in its socket, would indicate a descent from some more ardent regions than the chilly clime of Ireland. The configuration of the countenance is also too lengthy, and its different organs raised too highly into relief not to induce the observer to suspect, that the possessor of these characteristics is a stranger, or at least an exception to the fair, fleshy physiognomies of his native land. There is indeed, an air of foreign formation about his whole aspect, which induces us to believe that the family of the Graves are not sufficiently long settled in Ireland to be formed according to the standard of the native beauty of that country."

I interpret this to be a sly dig at the fact that the Graves family was one of those who came over with Cromwell.

"After passing through four or five generations more, they may possibly arrive at that honourable distinction, and appear as indigenous products of the soil. Dr Graves, however, has excited much attention, and strong hopes of eminence in the profession, since his appointment in the School of Physic. A course of study to which Dr Graves has fitted himself for this purpose, in some measure justifies these anticipations. Having exhausted our British Schools, he visited the continental seminaries and came home deeply impressed with a conviction of the superiority of their system of medical education, and with the determination of carrying it into effect in his native country. An opportunity soon presented itself for the accomplishment of this design, in an appointment to the Meath Hospital on his return. An attempt was accordingly made, but, with all his care, it has not, we understand, turned out a very successful experiment. Something was certainly done, for which he is entitled to the gratitude of all who take an interest in the improvement of medical education."

Erinensis goes on to say how: "Dr Graves still persists with most praiseworthy perseverance, in the prosecution of his design, and has, we are told, relinquished, in great measure his private practice, since his election to a professor's chair, that he might have more leisure to follow up his favourite pursuits. Such a disinteredness, at least, indicates that platonic affection for science which generally coexists with the power of extending its boundaries. His manner, indeed, during his discourse, struck us as being in perfect harmony with the enthusiasm of his disposition, and his love of communicating as well as of cultivating science. He passed on to the Professor's chair with an alacrity of motion, and opened on his audience in a tone of impassioned perusal from a manuscript which, to persons accustomed to less enthusiastic modes of address, and unacquainted with his own warm temperament, might be painfully startling. His countenance, naturally expressive of much latent emotion, even in a state of quiescence, when thoroughly excited, as it then evidently was, by the working of his feelings, together with the accompaniment of a husky, sepulchral voice, strained to its highest pitch, and let loose on his audience without much regard to modulation, struck us, we confess, with a degree of surprise, a little too electric to be agreable. Desire to impress the truth of his opinions on his spectators was obviously too powerful to be restrained by his taste and his judgement, for, during the whole of his discourse, he swept over the aching senses of his auditory in a whirlwind of enunciation, exhibiting all the tumult of a storm, without its grandeur or its force."

Erinensis never fails to poke fun at the foibles of the lecturer for he goes on to say of Graves: "he dealt too, pretty largely in those flowers of rhetoric, or elaborate figures of speech, so common to Irish writers, but which, in his inexperienced hands appeared to us to have been no other than 'potato blossoms'; and by way of being sublime, alternately passed from earth to heaven, now grubbing from the one, and next soaring among the prodigies of the other."

It has to be remembered that Graves' father had been a brilliant preacher as a young man in the churches of Dublin and no doubt in those days young Graves, with his brothers and sisters, had sat every Sunday in the family pew and picked up some of his father's oratorical skills.

So we have a picture of a young man, he was just over thirty-two years old, of swarthy countenance and black hair, with a strong aquiline nose and flashing eyes, who was a good lecturer and was always bursting with energy. He had a deep voice which he used to excellent advantage. He was extremely keen on research and observation of all kinds and did not give the demands of his private practice a high priority. Undoubtedly he was impetuous and his outspoken comments, often uttered without much regard for tact, landed him in hot water and made a number of enemies. He was a courageous person but never self seeking and had hardly been appointed to the staff of the Meath Hospital when he volunteered and went off to Galway to be in the thick of a major typhus epidemic. His intimate knowledge of the clinical patterns of typhoid and cholera was obtained first hand, and such exposure has always carried a significant risk of contracting and even succumbing to infection which indeed was what happened to a number of his colleagues.

The Gibson affair
Let us turn now to the Gibson affair as I shall call it. Robley Dunglison was a distinguished American medical educator who was persuaded to go as Professor of Medicine to the University of Virginia in 1833 when he was thirty-five years old. He had been born in England in the Lake District and qualified in Edinburgh. He spent most of his life as Professor of Medicine at Jefferson College in Philadelphia and finding Graves' published lectures on Clinical Medicine particularly valuable he wrote to him. Graves replied as follows:

9 Harcourt Street. Dublin
1st October 37

My dear Sir,
I, this day, received your letter, and am very glad indeed to find, that you approve of my Lectures. The Lectures, published this year in the *London Medical and Surgical Gazette,* are very correctly printed, and were sent by myself to that journal. I have detected only one important typographical error; viz at pg 258—in the 13th lecture on paralysis; 21st line of right column, read health instead of breath—I shall feel much flattered by your reprinting these twenty lectures. I shall willingly purchase a dozen copies from you, and pay the money to Longmans and Co. Booksellers, Paternoster Row, London, from whom your correspondent there can get the money. You will perceive that I have long adopted the opinion, lately put forward with great ability in the *American Journal* by Dr Gerhard, that the Maculated fever of Ireland is different from the so named Typhus of Paris. It is necessary to specify this. It is a great satisfaction to us here, to observe the progress our brethren in the States are making in all the Sciences, and especially the Medical. I always feel much pleasure in paying attention to physicians and surgeons of your country, who visit us, and, lately, have had the pleasure of seeing two eminent men, Dr Warren of Boston and Dr

Ludlow of New York. When any of your friends visit Dublin I shall be glad to have an introduction from you by them.

Yours very truly,
Robt. J. Graves.

Robert Dunglison then went on to record in his diary that: "I did not however, give many letters of introduction to him, especially after the visit of Dr Gibson, of the University of Pennsylvania, who gave great offence to Dr and Mrs Graves, and more especially to the latter—as I have been informed—by the notice which he gave of them and their establishment in the *Rambles in Europe,* which he published on his return. Soon after this, I introduced Dr Moreton Stille of this city to Dr Graves; who informed me on his return, that the observations of Dr Gibson had given so much offence, that a friend of his in Dublin advised him not to present his letter of introduction. He did so, however, and, although nothing could be more polite to him than Dr Graves, yet he could not help observing, at table, the constrained manner of Mrs Graves towards him. How much is it to be deplored, that the rashness and impropriety of one individual should mar the enjoyment of so many right minded persons, who may come after him."

William Gibson's book *Rambles in Europe in 1839* was published in 1841 and in it he characterised Graves as a man of "humour, high spirits, and quizzical propensities, peeping and prying into every hole and corner.... cracking jokes with the patients or pupils, or old women... too fond of analogy and drawing conclusions from solitary facts." Perhaps there is some truth underlying Gibson's unkind observations, but he must have been a difficult visitor for he went on to give even greater offence in Edinburgh and was a thorn in the side of the university authorities back home in Philadelphia.

Wilde's portrait of Graves
It was in 1839 that the distinguished eye and ear doctor, William Wilde, father of Oscar Wilde, was invited by the editor of the *Dublin University Magazine* to write a pen portrait of Graves for the Journal. It was to be one of a series which was planned to last some years, and the articles did in fact survive for many years covering most of the city's distinguished citizens. They were all published anonymously and many of them were illustrated by pen and ink sketches done by Charles Grey who was a Fellow of the Royal Hibernian Academy; his portrait of Graves is particularly attractive. The originals of these sketches, including the one of Graves, are now housed in the National Art Gallery of Ireland in Merrion Square.

It so happened that the editor of the Journal, M'Glashan, who was also a well known publisher in the House of Curry and

Company, was a good friend of Graves and so he approached him directly and asked if he would sit his 'portrait'. Graves agreed but only with reservations. "On two conditions only will I consent" he said. "First that Sir Philip Crampton and Henry Marsh [who were both leading physicians in Dublin at that time] appear before me; and, secondly, that my friend and pupil, Wilde writes my memoir." This modesty on Graves' part was typical of the man said his friend Stokes. The choice of Wilde was of course excellent because they had not only been close colleagues for some years, but they had been boyhood friends and Oscar Wilde's uncle, William Wilde's brother, had coached Graves for his entry into Trinity. Wilde was three years younger than Graves and their homes, together with that of their mutual friend William Stokes, were all close together in Merrion Square and they often visited each other socially. There is an amusing and very early photograph of William Stokes pouring out a glass of beer from a bottle for Wilde who stands beside him, taken at a party in Merrion Square.

Biographical sketches of living individuals usually present problems. It is recounted that while they were in manuscript form, some of the earlier 'portraits' which appeared in the *University Magazine* had been allowed to be reviewed by 'admiring friends' and as a result a good deal of alteration had gone on which was not always to the liking of the subject of the memoir and certainly not to the editor, because it delayed publication. It was for this reason that Wilde and M'Glashan did not let Graves or any member of his family or friends see the article before it appeared on the first of February 1842. We know all these intimate background details about the production of the memoir because they appeared in a foreword to a reprinting of it some twenty years later, in 1864, after Graves had died. By then Wilde had been knighted and was also able to declare himself the author of what originally had been an anonymous publication. Wilde also commented on the graphic pen and ink sketch by Charles Grey RHA. "It was", he said "very like the man in feature, figure, dress and attitude as all those who can remember him twenty-two years ago can attest, but it lacks the searching gaze, the animated expression and bright piercing eye, which no illustration can ever pourtray."

Wilde went about his task of biographer with his usual thoroughness. He wrote to Graves and said that he would like the facts and dates of his career to ensure his account was correct. Graves who was then just forty-three years old, unfortunately tied Wilde's hands, he sent him a single sheet of foolscap paper with what he wished to be included, adding that outside the circle of his strictly professional career he did not desire to appear. Now Wilde was an old friend and neighbour and in the past had heard Graves retelling some of his exploits when as a young man he had travelled round

Europe, so naturally he asked him to authenticate some of those anecdotes. For example he asked him about the well known story of the near shipwreck in the Mediterranean which he had often heard him recall. Graves replied rather brusquely: "Do not mind any of these things; do not say anything about the little tailor and the crazy ship. It is true that I saved my life on the occasion you refer to; but all I want now is to save the lives of others, especially good Irishmen." Naturally Wilde was as good as his word and so apart from referring to the vigour of Graves' intellect and untiring industry, and his extraordinary brilliant academic career we learn very little about the man as a man, but much more about his work in Ireland and a little about his travels, but most of all about his academic successes. This response to Wilde's request for information is so atypical of the ebullient young Graves of a few years before

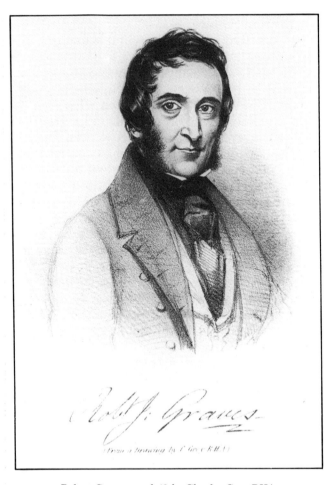

Robert Graves aged 43 by Charles Grey RHA.

that it is clear that by the year 1839 something had started to change his character. Perhaps this was the very beginning of that depression and introspection which overcame him in his later life. We hear much more of this in the next fourteen years.

Despite these restrictions which Graves imposed upon him, Wilde still wrote between nine and ten thousand words which duly appeared in the February issue with the charming portrait by Grey. Wilde must have thought highly of what he had written because he himself paid to have it reprinted twenty years later. Wilde, having sketched in Graves' upbringing, education and triumphant progress through Trinity and so to his three years in Europe, then gives his assessment of him as Professor of the Institutes of Physic as his title then described him.

"As a lecturer Professor Graves was endowed with peculiar capabilities. To a remarkable person he added great powers of arresting attention in the very outset of his discourse, which by an almost startling impressiveness he maintained throughout; his ideas were conveyed in a bold, fluent and classic style; in his language he was always forcible and elegant, and though frequently eloquent he never sacrificed his subject for flowers of rhetoric, or lost sight of his text in the froth of metaphor; for whether discussing the investigations of others, or detailing the results of his own enquiries, he ever manifested the same critical acumen, the same powers of the same piercing analysis. But higher and nobler far, we rejoice to say, that with the privileges he enjoyed he forgot not—both in his lectures and his addresses to the students, and in the presence of his professional brethren, whenever opportunity offered—to give the glory where glory is alone due, to speak the word in season; and while he taught his hearers what life does, and where it ends, he likewise led their minds to contemplate with gratitude the divine source from whence it sprung: in his own beautiful and expressive words:

"To create life is the attribute of God: to preserve life is the noblest gift man has received from his Creator. Life and death are involved in an eternal struggle; they succeed; they alternate, they displace, but never annihilate each other; they fill the world with their strife, but it is a strife where the antagonists contend like day and night, each chasing, but never overtaking each."

Wilde quotes extensively from this particular lecture of Graves with which he opened his course on physiology, ranging widely over everything from astronomy to theology. Such prose which was beloved of the Victorians is quite unfashionable today, but if one is prepared to pick out the facts there is much to ponder over. Wilde also tells of his contributions to the knowledge of acute fevers and their spread, the lymphatic system, nutrition and much else. We are told about his later travels in Europe: how he spent the summer of 1828 at the Charité and St Louis Hospitals in Paris, and the summer of 1829 in Hamburg. He recounts how with Dr Kane he founded the *Dublin Journal of Medical Science* which first appeared in 1832. He concludes with listing some of the publications of Graves' works in America and the translations into French, German and Italian.

Graves remembered posthumously

We are fortunate in having these two very different accounts of Graves and his work, written during his life-time. There are a number of biographical sketches which appeared after he was dead, but they have to be looked at in the knowledge that they are retrospective and coloured by the authors' later and mature consideration of what the man had been like. These all need to be considered as a whole after first reviewing the rest of his achievements. At this juncture, however, I believe that it is useful to recall some of the things which his closest friend, William Stokes, had to say about him in the very revealing prologue to the posthumous publication of 1863, his *Studies in Physiology and Medicine,* in which he was much more forthcoming about his old chief than Wilde was allowed to be. In temperament and character, Stokes was the perfect complement to Graves and this may in part account for their close friendship. Stokes came from a distinguished medical and academic family, well to do, and closely connected for many generations with Trinity. He was rather retiring and shy. Graves on the other hand needed the income which he earned from his private practice to pay his way. He was by nature somewhat extrovert, a forceful speaker, he also possessed considerable histrionic talent. Stokes was originally a pupil of Graves, indeed he was his favourite pupil, and subsequently became his junior colleague. His character was such that he never desired to usurp his senior's limelight. Stokes appears as a very gentle person in his portraits. This is how the pupil described his master:

"He had at once a warm and sensitive heart, and ever showed lasting and therefore genuine gratitude for the smallest kindness, loving truth for its own sake, he held in unconcealed abhorrence all attempts to sully or distort it; and he never withheld or withdrew his friendship from any, even those below him in education and social rank, if he found in them the qualities he loved, and which he ever admitted to honour.

"As bearing on this point, it is to be remarked, that his love of civil and religious liberty, often ardently and fearlessly expressed, led men of limited views to think him imbued with the doctrines of continental liberalism; yet he was, in principle, a thorough monarchist." Further on he continues thus: "it is to be observed that as his mind was open and unsuspicious, he, occasionally, fell into the error of thinking aloud without considering the nature of his audience, and of letting his wit play more freely, and his sarcasm in defending the right, cut more deeply than caution might dictate.

"This outline of the character of Graves at the commencement of his public life throws light on many matters relating to his subsequent career, and it is important to note that the world never spoiled him, so that he preserved most of the youthful, and all the kindly and better qualities of his mind up to the hour of his death."

This generous, warm, indeed loving portrait by Stokes of his old friend and chief tells us almost as much about Stokes as about Graves. Stokes was a very gentle and rather quiet individual and I believe this appraisal, made some ten years after Graves had died, overlooks much of the cantankerous and introvert side to his character which developed in his latter years. Those years when he was estranged from his wife, retired from his chair of medicine and from his honorary consultant post at the Meath and stopped writing for the journals.

Chapter 11

The Four O'Clock Lectures and Sir Patrick Dun's Hospital

If it really is possible to become an addict to hard work then this is what Graves became and it is still difficult to see how he achieved so much in every twenty-four hours. In modern jargon he would undoubtedly be dubbed a workaholic. As young Dr Guinness recalled, he was doing early morning rounds with his housemen by candlelight and later in the day he never failed to turn up in time to take his students on their teaching visit to the wards. He was greatly in demand for consultations in private and indeed he needed all the income he could raise at this stage of his career for he eventually had a family of six children, a large town house and a wife who liked to make a splash and entertain the leaders of society. Yet despite all this and the daily round to visit the sick in their homes he managed to go at precisely four o'clock every day, during term-time, to Sir Patrick Dun's Hospital and give a lecture—and what lectures they were! Their preparation alone would, for ordinary mortals, have taken up the rest of the twenty-four hours.

Stimulating and wide-ranging lectures

A hospital record says that the attendance did not fall below 140, and Sir William Wilde, who wrote his pen portrait, described the impact these lectures made:

"We well remember the stimulating effect the lectures of Dr Graves had upon the minds of the students such as we have described; who, at four o'clock, visited Sir Patrick Dun's Hospital to hear him. Then all weariness was forgotten—all langour vanished; the notebooks were again resumed—the attention that had already flagged at an earlier hour of the day, was aroused by the absorbing interest of the subject, and the energy of the lecturer; nay more; the noisy bustle usually attendant on the breaking up of a lecture was exchanged for discussions upon subjects treated upon or eager enquiries of the professor for the solution of difficulties—and the freshness of the morning again came over the exhausted student's mind."

He goes on to say: "Many of the introductory courses to these beautiful lectures, which included, among other subjects equally attractive, the infinity of life, the physical history of man, the doctrine of modern metaphysics—the physiology of the senses, the influence of physical agents affecting life, the wise provisions of nature for adapting life to every clime and quarter; language, electricity, intellect and instinct, medical statistics, food, and the connection between mind and matter are some which formed the material for his discourses one year, and pathology and therapeutics the next. Many were published in the *London Medical and Surgical Journal* between 1832 and 1834."

These rather flowery encomiums of Sir William Wilde, typical of a style prevalent in the 1840s, do in fact refer to a remarkable tour-de-force by Graves. I have on the desk beside me a tattered copy of the book entitled *Studies in Physiology and Medicine* by Robert James Graves edited by Stokes in 1863, just ten years after Graves died, and published as a memorial to the author by his brother the Revd Graves and William Stokes his old pupil and colleague at the Meath. The book is dedicated to the well-known Paris physician, Trousseau, and contains twenty physiological essays and twelve miscellaneous ones, the latter on a variety of subjects, from the spread of Asiatic cholera to some peculiarities of the skeleton in hunchbacks. The essays make fascinating reading today and many passages show that Graves was already formulating ideas which were not to be accepted for many years to come. His views on the lymphatic system were prophetic and his knowledge of diet and metabolism well before its time. The breadth of his reading and his catholic approach to the opinions of others, due in large measure to his travels all over Europe, which he continued each summer vacation for many years, are at once apparent. I am reminded as I read them of that latter day medical essayist, Lewis Thomas the American pathologist, in his 'Notes of a Biology Watcher' which have so often graced the pages of *The New England Journal of Medicine.*

A philosophical approach to the sciences

Here are some brief notes on a few of the lectures. In 'The Ubiquity of Life' Graves looked at the philosophy of one trying to 'understand' the world through the eyes of a biologist cum palaentologist cum naturalist; he was himself the complete polymath. He quotes from the work of Humboldt, Parry and Scoresby, who were contributing to the scientific literature of the day, as well as experiences from his own travels, to review the extraordinary spectrum of living creatures. The nineteenth century was a glorious period of scientific discovery in both the world of physical phenomena and of natural history. He had obviously used a microscope and gives good accounts of infusoria, algae and other animalcules. He was extremely well informed on a very wide spectrum of scientific matters of all kinds and this particular period, spanning the 1820s and 1830s, was one of much philosophical speculation about all the newly discovered biological and physical knowledge, collected from every corner of the globe.

Graves had much of the same kind of knowledge at his finger tips, such as the existence of marine fossils in the mountain valleys, growth of coral reefs and adaptation of living organisms to their environment as had Charles Darwin a few years later when he formulated his theory of evolution. Indeed Darwin, who was born sixteen years after Graves, was only persuaded to publish his great work *The Origin of Species by Means of Natural Selection* in 1859, some twenty years after he had first entertained it, as a result of a letter from Alfred Russel Wallace, who had come to almost identical conclusions after his work in the Malay Archipelago. No soi-disant physiologist that I can recall ever painted on so broad a canvas as Graves. The second lecture was entitled 'The Position of Man in the Scale of Life' and Graves with his thorough grounding in human embryology and anatomy, and his excellent grasp of comparative anatomy, comes near to formulating modern views on evolution, but then veers off to consider the importance of the five senses in providing information upon which the intellect can expand. He quotes fascinating examples of individuals born without one or more of their sense organs.

The biological response to physical changes
'The influence of Light' reviews the important part which light plays in metabolism in plants and he is particularly attracted by things which can survive in darkness, such as those that live in caves and deep in the ocean. In another thought provoking sally he goes on to give assessments of pressure, in pounds per square inch, on the top of Mont Blanc and at ocean depths of 100 and 1000 fathoms. He talks of the condor, that most magnificent of birds which can dart from the summit of Mount Chimborazo, one of the highest peaks in the Andes, to sea level—a change in barometric pressure of twelve inches of mercury to one of twenty-eight inches. How this can be explained in physiological terms still remains a mystery to most of us! This leads logically to the whale and its diving, he quotes from Scoresby on this, from Priestley on oxygen and from a multitude of other authors in many languages. It is not so surprising that students, of all ages, in Dublin flocked to hear him talk. I certainly would have been there.

In talking about phosphorescence, Graves is at his macabre best. He recalls how as a medical student he accompanied what he refers to as 'resurrectionary' expeditions to the grave-yard and noted the luminous appearance produced by the adhesion of phosphorescent matter to the old coffin boards which were turned up in opening the grave. He also remarked that when he was a teacher in the School of Anatomy at Park Street, "bodies presented, for one or two nights, a very singular and somewhat startling appearance, being covered all over with a phosphorescent effulgence." He goes on to talk of the brilliant phosphorescence in the sea due to Noctiluca, which, in the tropics, can look like liquid fire on the boat's side, and concludes with reports of similar appearances in mammalian eyes and plants.

There are similarly exciting lectures on the effects of temperature and the adaptation of the animal and vegetable kingdom to extremes of hot and cold. He refers to the forced feeding of geese in Strasbourg which are kept in artificial heat to produce the enormous liver used to prepare paté de foie gras and goes on to comment "How slight the difference between the morbid phenomena displayed in the post-mortem of a city feaster and the autopsy of an overfed goose." It is good to see an example of his humour, but as usual it always carries a sting in its tail. There is a long dissertation on electricity in relation to plants and animals. I cannot refrain yet again from quoting one of Graves' own remarks, remembering that this lecture was given in the 1830s. "Acupuncturation, in the common meaning of the term, has long been in use among the Chinese, and particularly among the Japanese, with whom the whole art of medicine seems to consist in teaching the names of diseases, and the number of needles to be employed in the cure of each. Its introduction into Europe is comparatively recent, and within my own memory. It has been found useful and its efficacy seems to have been very considerably increased by passing an electrical current along the needle". Today, more than a century and a half later, acupuncture is once again causing a stir in the western world.

An anthology of contemporary advances
Graves reviews a mass of fascinating information from the psychology of witch hunting in Salem to the instinct which leads to fighting in animals and human beings. He recalls Blumenbach's work on classifying different varieties of the human race and goes on to elaborate the theme with his own views on anthropology. He offers a thoughtful review of rhythm in biological systems, rhythm appears to be a fundamental quality of the universe. The hair, the skin, diet and nutrition, giants and dwarfs and theories of hearing and tactile sensation are all looked at in the light of recently published work, a veritable anthology of 'Recent Advances'. Stokes, for good measure, in his editorial capacity added to this retrospective collection of Graves' works a reissue of some of his most acclaimed writings, such as the article on the progress and contagion of Asiatic cholera, the workings of the lymphatic system and Dr Oppenheim's account, translated from the German by Graves, of life in Turkey.

Sir Patrick Dun's Hospital
These lectures which I have briefly touched on here, were originally

delivered, together with many others, in Sir Patrick Dun's Hospital. This building erected between 1803 and 1816 still exists, largely as Graves knew it, with its imposing entrance hall and fine staircase; the semicircular lecture theatre, which in those days was a great innovation in a hospital, has been twice rebuilt. It was one of the first purpose-built university hospitals to be put up in the British Isles and its characteristically Irish origins deserve a mention in their own right.

Patrick Dun, by whose name the hospital is known to this day, was born in Aberdeen in 1642, the son of a dyer, and attended the Medical Faculty of Marischall College of which his uncle was Principal and also Dean. He then travelled round Europe, studied and became a Doctor of Physic of the University of Valentia, which today is the French city of Valence on the river Rhône. He also received doctorates from Oxford and Dublin, and eventually settled in the latter city. By the age of thirty he had a huge practice and five years later, having been elected a Fellow of the Royal College of Physicians of London, in the days when it only had fourteen Fellows in all, he returned home and took an active part in the affairs of the Irish College of which he was elected President in 1677 and on numerous occasions thereafter. He also became a member of Parliament and married into one of the most distinguished families in Ireland. For his services to medicine he was knighted. Since Trinity refused to allow Catholics to become Fellows of the Irish College, he used his influence with the Lord Lieutenant to have a new charter passed based on that of the London College which did not discriminate against race or creed.

His only son and heir died at the age of three so he left his estate to his wife and at her death it went to the College of Physicians to be used to provide salaries for three professors to teach in the Medical Faculty of the University. The money accumulated far faster than it could be spent and there were endless legal wrangles about its disposal, even before, but especially after his widow died. The lawyers must have found the whole affair very profitable indeed. There then appeared on the scene Edward Hill who was both Professor of Botany and Regius Professor of Physic; his portrait catches your eye as you enter the lecture hall of the College of Physicians, he looks unhappy and was reputedly cantankerous. Hill had the idea of using money from the bequest to create a botanical garden for the medical students. In those days the study of medicinal plants, their properties and methods of extracting them formed a large part of the students' curriculum. However Robert Perceval, the physician who held the Professorship of Chemistry at Trinity lobbied for the money to be used for a teaching hospital. There have always been a multiplicity of small hospitals in Dublin and the students spent much time travelling round the city for their bedside instruction. The subsequent controversy does neither contestant much credit, but Perceval won the day although one has to admit that at that time Hill's proposal was a very reasonable one. Today, by contrast, the use of plant extracts has been almost completely replaced by man-made pharmacological compounds and the teaching or university hospital is at the hub of medical education. Thus in the long term Perceval had made the right decision.

The complete hospital was not opened until 1816 when Graves was just beginning his clinical years as a medical student at Trinity, it made a great impression on him as did its creator Robert Perceval who became his friend and hero, although of course many years his senior. The building itself is planned on the grand scale as one looks at the façade, being as much a monument to the memory of Sir Patrick Dun as a hospital for the instruction of the Medical Faculty of Trinity. In the event it seems completely appropriate that Graves should have given his lectures in the splendid setting of Sir Patrick Dun's amphitheatre.

Graves as Author

Graves wrote clear and unambiguous prose with a great command of the English language and his grammar was impeccable. Well versed in the classics, he could rarely resist inserting a neat and apposite quotation in Latin to illustrate a point. As a young man he tended to overdo this and some of his early letters home during his travels in Europe are at times constructed in a rather stilted manner, but it has to be remembered that at the time he was addressing his old teachers and no doubt thought that this would impress them, as would the classical quotations with which he larded the text. He quickly abandoned this trait and as soon as he was standing on his own feet as a consultant at the Meath Hospital, and a teacher in the Park Medical School, he adopted a clear style of exposition that never deserted him. He started contributing papers to the medical journals almost as soon as he returned from his travels in 1821 and for the subsequent twenty years they poured from his pen, the climax being in many ways his major treatise on Clinical Medicine which was to become a standard work on treatment all over Europe in its various translations, as well as in North America. His letter writing was always in fluent English; if he had a fault it was his occasional lapse into sarcasm which, on occasion, undoubtedly caused great offence.

Clinical reports

The medical writings covered a wide range of subjects and fell into several very different categories. By far the largest group was that containing articles on clinical matters, many of these were reports, or were based on reports, of individual patients whom Graves had seen in hospital or private practice. All through his career he was in great demand for a second opinion on patients with difficult problems and because of his clinical experience and very wide knowledge of the medical literature, which he constantly refreshed by reading journals as they appeared and translating German ones into English, he was the ideal choice. For example, he provided the first ever description of angioneurotic oedema, that distressing form of generalised urticaria or nettle rash, a quarter of a century before Dr Quincke of Kiel by whose name it is generally known today. Perhaps the fault lay in the fact that few French or German doctors at that time read the English language medical journals. The next group of his writings were those that were primarily physiological and were based on his lectures to the medical school in Park Street and at Sir Patrick Dun's Hospital. Some of these were printed first in Dublin but the majority appeared, either as reprints or *de novo,* in the *London Medical and Surgical Journal.* A miscellany of these which were published posthumously have already been briefly commented upon.

The three journals to which he originally sent his papers were the *Transactions of the Royal Irish Academy,* the *London Medical Gazette* and the *Edinburgh Philosophical Journal,* but he clearly needed a suitable local outlet for his medical writings and so Graves, with the great assistance and drive of his friend Dr Kane, founded the *Dublin Journal of Medical Science.* Kane was born in 1809 and having studied medicine at Trinity eventually became Professor of Chemistry there and later President of Queen's College Cork and the Royal Irish Academy; he was just the man to partner Graves in such a project. Graves was fascinated by the patterns of spread of diseases, today he would be called an epidemiologist. His interest in this stemmed from the days he spent with Hufeland in Berlin who was one of the founders of the science. It was growing expertise in epidemiology which contributed to the recent worldwide elimination of the scourge of smallpox. Graves made a particularly interesting and original observation while working in the city of Galway. Today, if you make your way to Nimmo's pier on the south bank of the river Corrib past South Park, you traverse an area known as the Claddagh. In Graves' day it was a separate fishing village of some 400 souls who took in no strangers and who had for their own consumption, plenty of fresh fish. They remained almost immune from the typhus epidemic and it was partly from this shrewd observation that Graves was able to point out that a good diet and isolation from infected individuals was the best way to contain an epidemic. It seems obvious to us now, but the majority of medical men in the early nineteenth century looked on typhus, typhoid, cholera and many other diseases as *not* being contagious.

A knowledge of German proved useful
Graves returned to Dublin from Galway and was immediately in the thick of things, consulting from his rooms, visiting the Meath Hospital early in the morning and delivering his daily lecture at Sir Patrick Dun's at four o'clock. Always on the look out for anything new in the field of medical science he had the added advantage of being able to read German as well as having access to all the British journals. This knowledge of German led him into at least one unusual task. When he had worked in Göttingen he had made the acquaintance of a Dr Oppenheim who subsequently went to serve in the Russian armed forces in Turkey. He was persuaded to enter the service of the Sultan and stayed on in that country for three years; in the early nineteenth century it was almost impossible for

a Christian to visit a Moslem country, far less work there. When Oppenheim returned to his native Hamburg he published a detailed account of his experiences. Graves, with his fluent German was so fascinated that he translated the text into English and summarised the main findings. It still makes good reading today. For example, there is an original and detailed account of the turkish bath, a communal affair, and what an important part it played in the health and social life of the men and women of Turkey. He described the various drugs that were in common usage and how circumcision and hernial repair were carried out. There is an intriguing description by Oppenheim of being present when an operation was being performed for a hernia, when he noticed that the encircling suture used by the surgeon inadvertently included the spermatic cord. Needless to say when Oppenheim pointed this out, the surgeon hotly denied it. He reported how polygamy was universal in Turkey at that time and eunuchs, who were boys castrated at six or seven years of age in Egypt, were regularly on sale in the market place in Constantinople, as Istanbul was then called. The extraction of teeth was in the hands of the barbers, who also brewed and sold coffee in the street. There are intimate glimpses into life in the harem which Dr Oppenheim obtained first hand when he was summoned by a Pasha to see a favourite wife who was critically ill. There are practical details on the preparation and use of cosmetics for which Turkish women were then and still are renowned. Turkey is to this day the world supplier of attar of roses.

Graves wrote on a wide range of subjects
Meanwhile Graves was contributing to the *Dublin Journal of Medical Science,* which from 1833 to 1836 was renamed the *Dublin Journal of Medical and Chemical Science;* no doubt the addition of 'Chemical' to the title was out of deference to Professor Kane who edited that part of the journal's contributions. Graves sent in an unending stream of case reports on a wide range of diseases which are listed in his bibliography. In other fields Graves demonstrated that he could write with skill and charm on an amazingly wide spectrum of nineteenth century science and so often brought to it that touch of originality which can still bring it alive today. For example he commented on the structure of the vertebrae of a young whale, its tender age being shown by the freely detachable epiphyseal plates; it had been stranded on the beach near Dublin. There is a paper on the sagittal suture in the skull of African natives and a splendid dissertation on the effects of the salinity of the water on life within and around the Dead Sea and the Great Salt Lake.

The Asiatic cholera pandemic
However, one of his outstanding contributions is a detailed, factual

and well reasoned description of 'The Progress and Contagion of Asiatic Cholera', an article which was reprinted with occasional additions in a number of places. His interest in this field having been kindled by Hufeland, it was fanned into flames by his collaboration with the mathematician Brinkley and then by his personal involvement in the typhus epidemic in Galway. This saga of the pandemic, since the whole world was eventually visited by the cholera, was written in 1848 to 1850 immediately after the appearance of the second and definitive edition of his two volume *Clinical Medicine* in which chapters 27 and 28 give a vivid and detailed account with dates and references of the route which the epidemic took in its spread both in and from Hindoostan (India) to Mauritius and Zanzibar and so on to South Africa, always by sea voyages. By land it spread by 1831 to the north of Russia and St Petersburg (Leningrad) and in the opposite direction through the East Indies to Hong Kong and Peking. In every case the date of its arrival and the likeliest means of transport by which it arrived is stated. All the European countries from Turkey, Greece and Hungary to Lithuania and Livonia (latterly Latvia and part of Estonia) in the north, are carefully documented, finally it arrived in England at Sunderland on November 4th 1832 by a direct sea route from Hamburg and next appeared in Edinburgh on January 27th 1833. The amount of work involved in recording all this data without the help of anything like a computer is almost beyond comprehension.

As Graves wrote: "It is exceedingly remarkable, how many of the great towns of England either escaped infection altogether, or were visited by only a trifling outbreak of the disease. Up to the 24th June 1832 (i.e. during a period of about eight months since its first appearance in Sunderland), the total number of cases throughout Great Britain, inclusive of London, amounted to only 14,796 and the deaths to 5,432. The disease, it is true, continued in many places to linger long after the above date, reappearing as an epidemic in some places in 1833 and 1834; in Great Britain and Ireland the cholera affected some 30,000 victims. In Ireland, particularly in Dublin and Sligo, the mortality was much greater than in England—an occurence which may, perhaps, be accounted for by "the bad diet of the Irish poorer classes and the crowded state of their dwellings". It has to be added that the New World did not escape. Cholera arrived in Quebec on about the 8th of June 1832.

Looking at the events of those days it is clear that Graves was hoping that with this essay he could more effectively combat the statement and policies of the Sanitary Commissioners in London that cholera was not contagious. They had circulated a notice that patients should be treated in General Hospitals and even went so far as to recommend that on the first appearance of cholera a placard stating this fact should be extensively circulated among the poor for the purpose of removing their apprehension! Fortunately in Ireland, the equivalent body, the Dublin Sanitary Association, under the direction of Sir Edward Burrough hurried a bill through the House of Commons setting up four isolation cholera hospitals in Dublin and similar arrangements throughout the country, which in practice worked well. Graves also poked fun at the proponents of the so called 'Fluvatile Theory' which maintained that cholera was always spread by rivers, they had gone so far as to say that it was by this route that the disease had travelled from Moscow to St Petersburg. Graves' riposte was "I would humbly offer as slight objection to the accuracy of this expression, that no river flows, or possibly could flow from Moscow to St Petersburg, as, if water attempted to accomplish the alleged journey, it would have on the way much uphill work". Graves was convinced, and tried with every shred of evidence which he could collect, to convince others that cholera was always contagious. When we remember that he was writing this many years before Pasteur and Lister postulated the bacterial basis of disease, and that it was not until the closing years of the nineteenth century that Koch demonstrated under the microscope some of the causal organisms—in this case the vibrio of cholera—Graves' work appears all the more impressive.

Graves' writings on current events
With such an enquiring mind it is not surprising to discover that Graves' interests were by no means confined to medical topics and we find him writing about current events, especially anything related to military undertakings overseas, and this was a time when the Empire was still expanding. Some of his articles are signed, but Stokes makes it quite clear that many important writings to which his name was not attached were contributed by him as leading articles in the public press. They are always distinguished by their careful preparation and a remarkable knowledge of history, geography, material resources and the prevailing political climate. One of these is of particular interest to us at the present day and that is his critique of the war in 'Affghanistan' which was in full spate at that time—spelling of foreign names has changed over the years, but hardly at all phonetically. In the nineteenth century it was the British who were struggling to master that country with the inhospitable terrain, so well suited to guerilla warfare, and it was the Russians who were aiding and abetting the local tribesmen. It could be said today that the boot was on the other foot. Graves wrote articles about it to the *Dublin University Magazine;* he first examined the state of English rule in India and then turning to Afghanistan he described the physical characters of the country and the tremendous strength of its natural defences. By that time the Cabool massacre had taken place

and General Nott was beleaguered in Candahar, Sale in Jellalabad and Palmer at Ghuznee. Thirteen thousand soldiers had already been killed in the Khoord Cabool Pass, but he pointed out that there was still a route into the country via 'Scinde'. The phonetic spelling of Indian and Afghan place names is rather attractive. He went on to review the pros and cons of further attack suggesting that the Russians were carrying on intrigues with the 'Affghan' chiefs with a view to invading India by that route. He makes it clear why such a move was unlikely to succeed because of the possibility of it uniting the native troops. This was indeed prophetic because later, in 1847, there was a great mutiny in the country.

A couple of sentences have such a suitable message for us today that here they are quoted in full:

"One thing is clear, that we must abandon Affghanistan the moment we have vindicated our tarnished honour, and rescued our beleaguered troops.

"God grant that we may be enabled to effect these objects, even though they cost us another seventeen millions, the sum already expended in this unholy war". Sentiments which I am sure are being echoed by the Russian leaders today.

Some of Graves' most valuable writings were on the functions of the alimentary tract, especially the stomach, and mention of this was made by his sponsors when he was elected a Fellow of the Royal Society. He also wrote extensively on diet and nutrition, especially the need to provide food for those who have no appetite for it, as for example those with high or prolonged fever or with cerebral disease. This seems to be the proper place to recall an anecdote which his friend Stokes loved to recall. It refers to an occasion when Graves was going round the hospital and when he entered the convalescent ward, he began to remark on the healthy appearance of some of the patients who had recovered from severe typhus.

"This is all the effect of our good feeding," he exclaimed; "and lest, when I am gone, you may be at a loss for an epitaph for me, let me give you one, in three words:

"He fed fevers"

Clinical Medicine
Graves' Magnum Opus

Graves' major written work in the medical field entitled *A System of Clinical Medicine* appeared in 1843 and although it was a large volume it was sold out in a few months. However, an interval of fully five years elapsed before the much revised second edition appeared and this was because Graves was so busy that he simply did not have time to devote to it. There are in addition some pointers to show that he was already beginning to suffer from that mental depression and physical inertia which was to overcloud his later years. When he eventually came to realise that he could not tackle the task single handed, he turned to Dr Moore Neligan, a physician who was on the staff of the London Hospital to help him. His choice of Neligan is interesting; Neligan's father and the rest of the family were well known to him in Dublin and the London Hospital was his very first port of call when he had set out as a young man and studied there with Dr Blizard. He must have enjoyed watching the career of his young protégé gaining such an eminent position. In a complementary way, it was a feather in Neligan's cap to be associated with such a prestigious publication. The second edition was eventually published in 1848, a year which proved to be a turning point in Graves' career for it was the year in which he retired from the Meath Hospital.

This second edition, which incidentally had now spread to two volumes, was a best seller on a worldwide scale for in addition to being extremely popular in the British Isles, it was translated into French, German and Italian and was also issued in the 'American Medical Library' in the USA. The French translation by Dr Jaccoud was published in Paris with a most flattering foreword by Professor Trousseau who was the leading physician in that city and bears a name honoured to this day in the field of neurology. Graves dedicated this second edition to the Right Honourable William, Earl of Rosse who was both President of the Royal Society and a friend. It was in the following year that Graves was made a Fellow of the Royal Society. Another interesting sidelight is introduced by Neligan in his editorial foreword where he explains that Graves was always in the habit of dictating all his work to a shorthand writer, which explains how his writings have a colloquial character, and I personally think that this gives them a warm and attractive style of presentation.

Lectures reprinted after 25 years

Some twenty-five years later, the New Sydenham Society which was founded in 1883, set about reprinting facsimile editions of many of the leading medical treatises which were out of print, but of historical value. One of their first ventures was to reissue Graves' *Clinical Lectures on the Practice of Medicine* and they prefixed it with an English translation of Trousseau's Introduction to the French edition. It is not a very good translation, but then they merely reprinted it from an old issue of the *Medical Times and Gazette*. This two volume edition is almost the only one to be found today and I have discovered it all round the world, usually on the top shelf of a medical library where it can be seen gathering dust. However, since Graves' reputation as a physician must depend on what is contained within its covers it is interesting to turn back the clock and see what in fact he wrote.

The limitations of nineteenth century medicine

To review the book in a proper perspective it is necessary to recall that a physician in the 1840s had none of the diagnostic aids on which his modern counterpart relies so heavily. No microbiology laboratory existed, for the bacteria and viruses had still to be discovered; there was no chemical pathology and even morbid anatomy was largely based on the naked eye appearances of the tissues. As for obtaining an electrocardiogram or EKG or an X-ray picture, the necessary technology was not to be invented for another fifty years or more. In addition, there is now assistance to be had from haematology, biological assays and all manner of scans. Graves was practising in an era when it was to be almost a hundred years before the first of the sulphonamides was available and as for penicillin, it was not until the mid 1940s before it first became usable clinically.

What then were the medicines which Graves could rely on to bring help to his patients? First and foremost and in common with all medical men for at least two thousand years there was opium. This in tincture form as laudanum could be given by mouth or by enema and Graves frequently refers to the latter route for administering all kinds of treatment to the very ill. There can be no doubt that over the centuries the use of opium and its derivatives, such as morphia and heroin, for the relief of pain and the induction of sleep, has been the single most important item in the armamentarium of a doctor. What else was there which he could turn to for help? Exceedingly few items on the apothecaries' shelves or in those intriguing little wooden drawers with their cryptic writing in black and gold, with which the walls of the dispensary used to be lined, could be relied on to produce a predictable and useful pharmacological effect.

Quinine, or Peruvian bark was good for ague, the word malaria was used at that time to describe the vapours which arose from swamps. Digitalis, the name given to the dried leaf of the foxglove was used in heart disease for swollen ankles and the more generalised oedema of dropsy, but Graves remarked how it was claimed to accentuate the difference in the pulse rate between standing and lying down. He quoted his own experiments in testing this and went on to quote Humboldt's work in which he said the frog's heart beat at twenty per minute when suspended, but at only nine per minute when horizontal. As an extension of this he quoted Baer who made the curious observation that in hatching eggs artificially, the chick *in ovo* soon dies if the egg is placed so that it lies on either end. Graves then suggested that this is why all avian eggs are oval because if they were round they might take up a position that was fatal for the enclosed embryo. He then proposed that research ought to be planned to find out why the human fetus is suspended upside down down *in utero* for such a position taken up after birth would soon be insupportable. Graves was always a stimulating and provocative thinker and teacher.

For the first half of the nineteenth century only a few chemical compounds were in regular use medicinally. Mercury was the mainstay of treatment for syphilis and much prescribed in the form of calomel by mouth or incorporated into an ointment which was rubbed into the skin, a new area being chosen each day. Arsenic was also used very widely without much idea of how it worked. Graves was particularly keen on the use of tartar emetic which is the double tartrate of arsenic and antimony which had originally been used by the Arabs to produce purging and vomiting and from whom its name is derived. Graves believed it softened and helped to detach the mucus from the tongue and the lining of the stomach. The remainder of the available medicines were vegetable decoctions of one kind or another, like tincture of squills for cough, which is still in use today in many proprietary preparations. As a child I loved oxymel of squills which I was given if I had a cough, it was a most attractive mixture of honey with an alcoholic extract of squills, those little bulbs which produce sheets of blue flowers on the Welsh cliffs in Spring. But, for the most part, prescriptions were empirical, it was sufficient to say that the great doctor so and so used it and that was reason enough. There were some other weapons in the doctors' pharmacopoeia, often dramatic in their use, especially from the patient's point of view, which are rarely seen today. Leeches were applied to reduce local swelling and in those days could be ordered for anything from a black eye to a stroke. Cupping was popular and its use is still seen occasionally on the continent of Europe, it is primarily a method of counter irritation. Most dramatic, and particularly from the relatives' point of view, was bleeding, in which a pint or more of blood was removed by opening a vein in front of the elbow, often using a traditional knife called a phlebotome. This

draconian step often did more harm than good, weakening still further a debilitated person, as was the case with Keats. However the doctor no doubt quoted Hamlet to good effect:
    "Diseases desperate grown
    By desperate appliances are reliev'd,
    Or not at all."

The general treatment of fevers

It is fair criticism to say that Graves, in treating his patients, used an immense number of substances, many of which have not stood the test of time. But, and this is his strength, he prescribed nothing without giving good reasons for doing so, although it is now clear to us that he was sometimes wrong, and he was always quite precise in his dosage and the duration for which the medicine should be given. Most important of all he took immense pains to discover the patient's background, both at home and at work, and tried to find out why they were sick in the way that they were. In addition he was probably the best informed and certainly the best read doctor in the Dublin of his day and a superb diagnostician. He believed, taught and practised that treatment of the whole patient was the basis of good medicine. The holistic approach is how it would be described today. Here are some of his particularly down to earth instructions in the chapter on 'The General Treatment of Fevers".

"Now when called on to treat a case of fever, there are several things which need your attention. In the first place, you should examine the state of the family arrangements. This is a matter which men are apt to overlook or treat as a matter of indifference, but in my mind it is of no ordinary importance, and should always be attended to. You should never, if possible, undertake the care of a case of fever where the friends or relations of the patient supply the place of a regular fever nurse. The mistaken tenderness of relatives, and their want of due firmness, presence of mind and experience, will frequently counteract your exertions and mar your best efforts. Affection and sorrow cloud the judgement, hence it is that very few medical men ever undertake the treatment of dangerous illness in the members of their own families. The sympathy which a nurse should have for her patient should be grounded on a general anxiety to serve, and a strict sense of duty, as well as a laudable desire of increasing her own reputation; it is, in fact, a sympathy analogous to that which should activate a physician.

"There are many nurses who are extremely attentive, but inexpert and injudicious, and their ill-judged attentions are frequently prejudicial to the patient. A fever nurse has a vast deal in her power; if an enema is to be administered, the patient will be much less disturbed and annoyed than if it were given by an unskilful person. The mere handling of a patient—the moving of him from one bed to another—the simple act of giving him medicine or drink—the changing of his sheets and linen—the dressing of his blisters—and a thousand other offices, can be performed with advantage only by an experienced nurse.

"If the patient is restless for instance, the ill-judged anxiety of his friends will most certainly prevent him from sleeping. They steal softly to his bed, draw the curtains, move the candle so as to make the light fall on his eyes, and wake him perhaps at the moment he is settling down to rest. If he happens to take an opiate, and they are aware of the nature of his medicine, they inform him of it, and his anxiety for sleep, conjoined with their enquiries, prevents its due operation. Hence when you prescribe an opiate, you should not in any case say anything about it; and it should not be administered in such a way as to lead the patient or his friends to expect decided benefit from it. It is only when I have to deal with prudent persons, that I break through my rule of concealing both the nature of the medicine and the results which I expect from its operation.

"The bedroom of a patient labouring under a fever should be well aired, but not what is termed thorough air; and it should, if possible, be a quiet back room away from the street. In the next place, it should be sufficiently large to hold two bedsteads conveniently; and you should order the attendants to have two well aired beds in readiness, from one of which the patient should be changed to the other every twelve or twenty-four hours, you can scarcely have an idea of the comfort this affords to a person in fever."

As one who has spent an unreasonable number of spells in hospital as a patient, the writer can confirm that a bed skilfully made is a considerable boost to morale, while one dreads the attentions of an inexpert nurse. To sit up in a bed with freshly laundered sheets and pillow slips is one of the few pleasures of life left for the sick. I have found it fascinating to read sections of a textbook on medical treatment written about 150 years ago. The common diseases we encounter today remain just as they were then; only the approach to them has changed, due to our new knowledge of physiology and pathology. I am glad to say that in some cases the treatment has improved vastly.

Another source of Graves' strength was in his approach to disease through the pathological changes which he was constantly seeing, and actively seeking, in the post-mortem room. For example in neurology many of the diseases are as little affected by treatment today as they were in his time. His accounts are often anecdotal but so frequently related to what he later discovered was the pathological basis of the physical signs. There is a wonderful lecture on apoplexy illustrated by two personal clinical accounts of patients together with the subsequent post-mortem findings. They read like the case reports of the Massachusetts General Hospital as published weekly, to this day, in the pages of the *New England Journal of Medicine*. He also makes it clear that often no explanation is found at autopsy or only one of those that are "sought with such avidity that they are always found".

He was proud to relate the story of a victim of chest disease whose condition of pyopneumothorax, which is the presence of both pus and air in the chest, was diagnosed by him with Laennec's stethoscope when it had only just been introduced as a diagnostic aid in chest disease. Lung diseases were very prevalent in those days and some sixty thousand people were dying annually in Britain from tuberculosis alone. He was a strong advocate of good food and fresh air as the best preventive for consumption as it was still called at that time.

Rheumatic fever was still particularly common though it seems to have disappeared in most countries in the last fifty years. Graves clearly distinguished it from gout by the response, or lack of it, to colchicum. He writes "Colchicum, if it does not afford relief in a short time and in moderate doses, there is no use giving it a further trial". He was keen on blistering, the use of mercurial ointment, warm baths, spa and hydrotherapy. His treatment of sciatica was empirical as all too often it still is today; he favoured cupping along the course of the nerve, morphia, and care in avoiding flexion of the back. It was, however, in the management of the acute fevers that he was able to call on his immense experience.

Graves devoted some 415 pages of his first volume to the treatment of fevers and they certainly constituted a major part of the work with which the nineteenth century physician had to contend. Today, when we have precise means of diagnosis in the laboratory and a wide range of antibiotic treatments available, we find it difficult to appreciate the preeminence of the fever problem in the mind of the doctor at that time. What were the fevers which Graves recognised and wrote about? The list is formidable: typhus, typhoid, cholera, yellow fever, scarlet fever, ague or malaria, and influenza. Measles, chicken pox and other acute infections of childhood are not given individual mention. No doubt when Graves was writing about yellow fever he must also have been seeing cases of what are today called hepatitis.

Treatment of typhus–the model for fevers in general
Typhus figures so largely in medical writings of the period when Graves was working, that it deserves special mention here. In developed countries it is something of a rarity and I personally, including many trips overseas, have never knowingly encountered a single case. It is caused by a Rickettsia organism transmitted by the body louse and is highly infectious. Typically it occurs among the overcrowded, uncleanly and particularly the underfed. The louse is found characteristically hiding in the seams of clothing. Typhus has always been a scourge of armies and in olden times followed in the wake of those civil disasters which led to destitution

and overcrowding.

Trousseau stated in the introduction that prefaced the French translation of Graves' *Clinical Medicine* that:

"Graves has devoted a great many lectures to typhus fever, which so cruelly decimates Ireland. It might be supposed at first sight, that the study of this portion of his work is not of much importance to us French physicians, who fortunately have not had to contend with the formidable malady in question; this is a mistake. All the precepts of the author upon the treatment of this pyrexia are so applicable to the severe forms of our typhoid fever, that we shall with the greatest advantage consult this remarkable work; moreover, the maxims related to the regimen have become the guide of the practitioners of all countries; it is they which now direct us in the treatment of putrid fever. And nevertheless, when he inculcated the necessity of giving nourishment in long-continued pyrexias, the Dublin physician, single handed, assailed an opinion which appeared to be justified by the practice of all ages; for low diet was then regarded as an indispensable condition in the treatment of fevers. Had he rendered no other service than that of completely reversing medical practice upon this point, Graves would, by that act alone, have acquired an indefeasible claim to our gratitude". I myself well remember as a child being told to eat up and I wonder how often others have been plagued by the maxim "Stuff a cold and starve a fever". It is significant that it is only in the last few years that there has been a worldwide programme to promote the use of salt and glucose in water for the treatment of typhoid and epidemic diarrhoea in infants and others in those epidemics which are such a plague in the third world, especially in times of famine.

Graves, although he wrote at such length on typhus was using it as the prototype for the treatment of fevers in general; many cases of fever diagnosed loosely as typhus may indeed have been typhoid, which in those days was endemic in much of Europe. Queen Victoria's consort, Prince Albert, died of typhoid fever at Windsor Castle, undiagnosed. Even today the disease can still provide a diagnostic puzzle. Trousseau was undoubtedly correct when he said that Graves' proposed epitaph 'He fed fevers' probably saved more lives than any other contribution he made.

The spread of epidemics

In his great work on Clinical Medicine, Graves devoted the first six chapters to general matters such as how to examine a patient and the pathology of inflammation, then chapters seven to twenty-nine are all about fevers and the first volume concludes with sections on joint diseases and those of the nervous system. Needless to say he lays great stress on the patterns of spread of epidemics throughout the world and also the factors governing the death rate. Some of the quotations he gives about living conditions are more reminiscent of

Dickens than a textbook of medicine. For example in discussing cholera he remarks that many of the 'great towns' of England escaped the epidemic or were only slightly affected and in the subsequent eight months the total number of cases was 14,796 with 5,432 deaths. On the contrary in Ireland, particularly in Dublin and Sligo the mortality was much greater than in England—"an occurrence" he says "which may, perhaps, be accounted for by the poor diet of the Irish lower classes, and the crowded state of their dwellings, it being well known that in the worst quarters of the city many families reside on the same floor, and frequently more than one in the same room". Graves then quoted from an article by Dr Elliotson in the *Medical Gazette:* "In London the greater part of the people are well fed, better fed than in any other part of the world; they eat more meat, and the flesh is of such quality as is scarcely to be found in any other country. Beside which they are better clothed and more comfortable; and instead of trashy wines they have good sound ale and porter, and malt liquor of all kinds. But in Paris the water the inhabitants drink is very bad; the people are crowded together, I know not how many families in a house, with little ventilation. The streets are narrow, the houses dirty; and the population live on what the Englishman considers trash, not roast beef and mutton, but all sorts of dishes made up of bread and vegetables, with a little meat boiled in water to colour it or give it a flavour; and drink not good beer, but thin wine." One begins to wonder if Dr Elliotson ever made a visit to Paris! How different today is the Englishman's opinion of his French host's gastronomy and cellar.

Graves continued by pointing out that the death rate in Paris was much higher than in London; 85 dying in a single day of April 1832. Cholera soon spread from England to Ireland, the first case being reported in Dublin on March 22nd and by the next month it had reached Belfast. However, it did not appear in Waterford and Wexford until July and August and Graves pointed out that at that time there was no direct connection by steam (railway) between Dublin and those cities, while a steamer plied twice a week to Cork where cases were first reported as early as April 12th.

Graves deduced from all these observations that cholera was contagious, a view that was not held universally at that time. He also quite correctly deduced that the main cause of death in the disease was the extreme loss of fluid in the stools, but his introduction of the use of lead acetate as a means of slowing up the diarrhoea, though ingenious, was ineffectual as we now realise. The more one reads this masterely work on Clinical Medicine, the more it becomes apparent how far ahead was his thinking compared to that of his contemporaries. Probably for this very reason he was not always a popular figure among the fellow members of his profession in Dublin.

Chapter 14

1846 Famine and the Corrigan Affair

The great famine which resulted from the blight destroying the potato harvest in the summer of 1846 brought to a head the problems which already existed due to maladministration, absent landlords, and the neglect of centuries. The peasants, and they really were peasants in the pejorative sense that the word is often used today, especially in the South and West of Ireland, lived largely in hovels from hand to mouth. There was little education and less food and the whole economy was based on the potato. Such grain as was grown was exported, it was far too expensive for agricultural workers to eat. Fishing had hardly been developed to provide an item of diet, this was as much due to ignorance of its potential as food as from the lack of money with which to buy boats capable of going out to sea. The disastrous famine of 1845 to 1850, so eloquently portrayed in Cecil Woodham-Smith's book *The Great Hunger* was the worst of a series of famines which had recurred over the previous 150 years and it was the 'fever' which accompanied the famine which actually caused the huge death toll.

William O'Brien, as head of the Department of International Health and Tropical Medicine recently reviewed the diseases which were primarily responsible for the high death rate in the potato famine and concluded that the prime killer was louse-borne typhus, followed by louse-borne relapsing fever, cholera, dysentery, smallpox, severe measles and typhoid, in that order. Today, smallpox has been eliminated from the list.

Graves was no stranger to famine or to epidemics of typhus, for when he was still a very young consultant physician at the Meath Hospital in 1823 he had volunteered to lead a group of relief doctors to help in an epidemic in Galway following the death of the doctor in charge and two of his successors. This epidemic also followed failure of the potato crop and the effects were worst in the country district of Connemara. The poor flooded into the city of Galway and the overcrowding combined with the great poverty and lack of food led to an outbreak of typhus with great loss of life.

There were to be further epidemics on a lesser scale before the disastrous one which followed the potato blight in 1846. During one of these in 1836 a fever specialist from Geneva, Dr Lambard, visited the main centres in England and Ireland and sent two communications to the *Dublin Journal of Medical Science* in the form of open letters addressed to Dr Graves. These letters are especially important to us for it has often been a criticism of Graves that he did not distinguish clearly between typhoid and typhus, but they clearly provide evidence that he was indeed correct. In the first letter, dated June 16th Dublin 1836, Dr Lambard pointed out that in the fever named typhus in Europe, when the body was examined post-mortem there was always a characteristic swelling and ulceration of the Peyer's patches of lymphoid tissue in the terminal ileum which is that part of the small bowel that empties into the large bowel and because of this, purges given to the patient usually had a disastrous effect, often leading to perforation of the small bowel, peritonitis and death. But when he attended post-mortem examinations in the fever hospital in Glasgow and the Meath and Hardwicke hospitals in Dublin, none had enlarged Peyer's patches. We know now that enlarged Peyer's patches are found in typhoid not typhus, so Graves was correct in his diagnosis of typhus in Galway.

The papular measles-like skin rash which Lambard reported in his Geneva patients was unlike the widespread rash with petechiae seen in Dublin. In addition, the typhus in Geneva rarely affected the nurses, doctors and students, but in Ireland six or seven percent of fever doctors died. In his second letter, Dr Lambard went on to say that he later visited fever hospitals in Liverpool, Manchester, Birmingham and London and found the fever just as contagious as in Ireland and only very occasionally were the Peyer's patches swollen. He concluded that the Dublin fever was typhus, typhus contagieux, fièvre des armées, fièvre des prisons, and was rarer in Liverpool, Manchester, Birmingham and London in descending order because it was conveyed thence by the Irish journeymen taking some days on the journey. He added that typhoid disease with large Peyer's patches did occur in Great Britain, accounting for one third of the patients in Glasgow and one quarter in London.

This splendid clinical and pathological distinction between typhus and typhoid made before the days of Pasteur and Koch and the subsequent discovery of the causative organisms, abundantly supports Graves' definitions of these diseases and it also shows what an accurate clinician he really was. It was a fellow countryman of Dr Lambard, the Swiss anatomist Johann Conrad Peyer who lived from 1653 to 1712, who first described the lympoid patches which are found in the lower reaches of the small intestine and enlargement of which is so characteristic of typhoid as opposed to typhus.

Epidemics follow famines
Where there is famine, there are epidemics and in Ireland in the 1840s, with its poor housing and little provision for personal cleanliness or sanitation, it was soon apparent that disease was overtaking the population in an alarming fashion. Typhus was the main offender; it has been the scourge of armies since prehistoric

times, and is spread by the body louse. The causative organism enters the louse when it sucks the blood of an infected person, and it is passed in the insect's faeces on to the skin where it soon gains access to the tissues via a scratch or by the mouth; the intense irritation of the louse bites guarantees scratching and infected material is picked up by the nails. It is also believed that at the height of an epidemic, the dried faeces of the louse may blow off the skin and the clothes in contact with it and, being inhaled, cause further spread of the infection. It is unusual to find lice on the skin except when taking their daily fill of blood, instead they cling to the inside of the clothing and typically lay their eggs along the seams. They thrive and multiply at the temperature of the body, but if this rises too high as in fever, or falls because their victim dies, they move on to the next provider of blood and thus spread the disease. Once the individual is infected, incubation takes place in five to fifteen days. The individual develops a headache, backache and shivering and then the temperature rises. Nose bleeds are common and a rash spreads over the body while the fever swings up and down and is often accompanied by delirium. In about three weeks the more fortunate patient begins to recover but unhappily many died during the 1846 epidemic, the virulence of the typhus usually increases as the disease spreads.

Many other disabling infections occur in a famine-struck community. Dysentery due to bacteria such as the Salmonella group, which cause typhoid and paratyphoid, are the main offenders, the death rate being highest among children who succumb to dehydration more swiftly than their parents. In the last few years the importance of providing water and nourishment to infants with dysentery, that is glucose and salt in water by mouth or by vein, has saved far more lives than any antibiotic, especially in the famine disaster areas of tropical countries. Once again this is eloquent testimony in favour of Graves' campaign to 'feed fevers'.

Foreign aid supplements the Irish health service
Now to return to the great potato famine of 1845. Potato blight, which is caused by the fungus *phytophthora infestans,* was no stranger to Ireland nor indeed to most countries in Europe; it had affected the crop on at least three previous occasions in the nineteenth century, but it was the suddeness and the completeness with which it destroyed virtually the entire crop in 1846 which led to widespread famine in an already impoverished community. The eye-witness accounts of what happened are heart rending and even in these days of disastrous famine in central Africa, are horrifying to contemplate.

Help came in the form of relief from England and America; the Society of Friends, or Quakers, including those in the USA, were swift and generous in their support. Thousands of families fled to the ports to emigrate, usually to America, but the death toll in these ships, which were often crowded and quite unsuitable to deal with outbreaks of infection, was alarming. Some overall idea of the magnitude of the loss to Ireland can be guessed from the census figures which showed a fall in the population from eight to six million in five years.

It must not be thought from looking at the horrific details that Ireland as a country had no social conscience. From the beginning of the nineteenth century a concerted drive was made by Government to augment what had usually been provided by voluntary subscriptions with building Free Dispensaries and there were 636 of these by 1845. It is true that the doctors who staffed them were sometimes not well trained and they were poorly paid for their services, but Ireland, over the centuries, has produced far more doctors than the homeland could afford to employ. As in England there had been a move to provide County Infirmaries and more than thirty were already in use, and then in addition the equivalent of the English Poor Law Institute or Workhouse Hospital had also appeared, there were more than a hundred of these. Naturally the beds would have been largely occupied before the 'plague' struck and soon the hospitals were all disastrously overcrowded; nothing spreads epidemics more effectively than overcrowding. Temporary huts and tents were erected in the grounds and efforts made to bring in more food. The basic ration was often 'stirabout', a porridge typically made from corn meal.

It has to be conceded that under the Prime Minister, Robert Peel, and the Parliament of the day, the country was seeing the results of almost half a century of real endeavour to provide Ireland with a basic national health service in advance of many other European countries. The damp climate and the poor nutrition, however, needed more than poor law hospitals and dispensaries to deal with them. Just as we have seen in Ethiopia in 1984 and more recently in the Sudan, the ravages of famine attracted aid from overseas, and the subsequent administration of this showed up the cracks in government and civil service to the alarm of the benefactors. But worse was to come, for professional pride had been piqued and two of the leaders of the medical profession, Graves and Corrigan met head on.

Corrigan's background
Dominic Corrigan was born above his father's shop in the Liberties in Dublin just five years after Graves. We owe a great debt to Eoin O'Brien for his discovery of the Corrigan papers and for the excellent biography he constructed from them in 1983 entitled *Conscience and Conflict*. It conjures up a picture of life in Dublin's

medical and political circles in the early nineteenth century as well as making Corrigan live again in its pages. Unlike the Protestant Graves family, the Corrigans were intensely Roman Catholic and therefore lacked the privilege of the Protestant ruling Irish community with its Trinity College, which by then had only just allowed the Catholics to take its degrees. However, his family was prosperous and ambitious enough to send him to St Patrick's College, Maynooth, which opened in 1795 as the first and foremost school for the education of 'nobility and gentry of Catholic persuasion'. He was a bright boy with a prodigious appetite for work and he started on his chosen career as apprentice to the physician and apothecary appointed to the college, who was also a general practitioner in the district. Young Corrigan then went to Trinity and attended for five years, using his vacations for further instruction in some of the other medical schools in the city. Then he proceeded to Edinburgh and graduated MD in 1825—a not uncommon practice in those days for an Irish doctor.

Thus Corrigan had none of the social advantages which Graves had when he qualified, but by sheer hard work and tenacity he gained appointment to the staff of the Charitable Infirmary in Jervis Street and eventually received international recognition for his work on heart disease and in particular aortic valve incompetence—even today all medical students are taught about Corrigan's pulse, the hallmark of the condition. Appointments to more prestigious hospitals followed and as he was an excellent teacher he was in great demand. With his increased earnings he started to visit clinics in France and Germany. Eventually he was being asked for advice by the Lord Lieutenant at the Castle in Dublin and, with a burgeoning private practice, he settled in a house at Number 4 Merrion Square, the most fashionable district in Dublin and very close to the houses of Graves and Stokes. Thus it was that when Parliament, goaded into activity by the famine, passed the Temporary Fever Act in 1846 and empowered the Lord Lieutenant to appoint Commissioners of Health to serve on a Central Board of Health, Dr Corrigan's name was added to those of Routh, who had been the Duke of Wellington's commissariat officer at the battle of Waterloo; Crampton, surgeon at the Meath Hospital; Robert Kane a distinguished chemist and doctor, and in addition, the Irish Poor Law Commissioner, Twistleton.

The Board had an impossible task. As the enormity of the disaster began to be seen, it tried to alleviate suffering by setting up temporary fever hospitals and appointing medical officers to them. This was indeed one of its statutory duties as stated in the Fever Act, as was also that of establishing the fees that should be paid for the services rendered. It was at this juncture that Corrigan made a mistake which was to damage his reputation in the public eye for the rest of his professional life. Corrigan recommended, and in fact it was he who attended the Board's meetings much more often than his colleagues, that the fever doctors should be paid five shillings a day, which was of course in addition to their ordinary salary. Dispensary doctors were only receiving an average of £71 per annum, but they had been given more than five shillings per day in the 1840 epidemic and this time the fever was much more lethal, many of them were dying after contracting the fever while looking after the sick.

Over a thousand doctors signed a petition to the Governor General protesting at this meanness and the newspapers, with one exception, took up the doctors' case and singled out Corrigan for their opprobrium. In England the *Lancet* considered that the members of the Board of Health should have resigned rather than be party to the award. At this point Graves entered the fray with a thirty page letter to the *Dublin Quarterly Journal of Medical Science* mainly directed at Corrigan. Graves, who had recently been President of the Royal College of Physicians and his colleagues on the Council were furious with the Government for not consulting them first. The Board were blameless, for Crampton was a past President and Kane was a Fellow. However Graves was quite correct in noting that "for during Sir Philip Crampton's absence in London and Sir Robert Kane's uniform non-attendance, Dr Corrigan was for many weeks the Board of Health and, consequently neither the College of Surgeons nor the College of Physicians was represented at that Board." Eoin O'Brien comments: "Had the doctor from the Liberties been rising a little too speedily for Graves' liking?"

Corrigan wisely did not reply to these criticisms but he did something that can only be interpreted as provocative and foolhardy; he chose this moment to apply to the Royal College of Physicians of Ireland for admission to their Fellowship. It seems extraordinary that he should have made this request at such a time. He already had many prestigious titles. For example he was a Fellow of the Royal College of Surgeons of London and when he had sat for this the examiners excused him from a *viva voce* examination because they recognised his outstanding contribution to knowledge of diseases of the aortic valve. In addition his colleagues had already elected him President of the Dublin Medico-Chirurgical Society, the most prestigious medical forum in Ireland. Surely he could have waited for a more opportune moment. Needless to say his application to the College of Physicians was blackballed.

Graves and Corrigan clash
There was also another and more personal reason for disagreement between Graves and Corrigan. Corrigan, when he laid down meas-

ures to control the epidemic of typhus proclaimed "no famine, no fever" and though in large measure this was true, his insistence on a single cause had disastrous consequences. With his firmly stated priorities he looked on time and money spent on preventing or containing the contagion as wasted. He simply did not believe that the beggars who roamed the south and west of Ireland were carrying the disease from place to place and Graves attacked him for his point of view. To quote Graves' own words: "The text put forward so authoritatively—'if there is no famine, there will be no fever'—prevented proper attention being paid to the real causes which produced and promoted the spread of epidemic diseases. The Irish epidemic had its origin in the congregating together of large masses of people at public works, the overcrowded workhouses and relief depots. Eagerness of impulse to apply relief continued with a total disregard of mode, and pestilence had followed the footsteps of benevolence and death wakened no suspicion of error. These measures were agencies of slaughter." These are the utterances of a very different Graves from the charming and brilliant young man who used to give the four o'clock lectures at Sir William Dun's Hospital.

Of course Graves was right, but he did rather overstate his case and his whole attitude was authoritarian. For instance, after a previous epidemic in 1818 two of the leading physicians of the day, Barker and Cheyne, had produced a report to the Government expressed in a much more balanced and moderate fashion. Barker and Cheyne stated in their report that there was no doubt that the famine was the prime cause since the epidemics which cropped up from time to time in Ireland always followed a failure of the main supply of food. They also pointed out that this was often lost sight of and the Government should take steps to avoid it in the future. They went on to say that even though the epidemics followed severe deprivation among the population, the fever was maintained by contagion operating on those predisposed by hunger and lacking in the habits of cleanliness. Those who argued against the contagious nature of typhus were entirely mistaken and were a danger to society—the spread of the epidemic was to a large extent due to movement of infected people from their homes and their subsequent crowding together. They also noted that clothes and bedding were vehicles of infection. They recommended that once there was evidence of spread of the fever there were measures that could be taken to contain it in much the same way as we observe with our international health and quarantine regulations today.

Graves' letter to the *Dublin Journal* would probably, if written today, have made him liable to be sued for libel, but it would have been a difficult case to try, for there was much truth in his allegations. He was never a tactful person, and on the whole he was merely giving expression to his own feelings and those of his fellow

Councillors sitting round the table at the Royal College of Physicians in Kildare Street. It serves however to draw attention to the change in character and outlook of the man who was now in his fifties, and judging from his portrait in a coloured daguerrotype, looking much older and unhappy.

Here is a letter reproduced from the *Dublin Journal of Medical Science* on the subject of cholera which is a good example of Graves' biting sarcasm and contempt for those who disregarded his soundly argued points of view:

"Letter on the Contagiousness of Cholera. By RJ Graves, MD
Merrion Square, October 16, 1848

Dear Sir,—In consequence of the appearance of cholera in England since my communication in the present Number of your Journal was printed, I beg leave to make the following observations on the progress of that disease:

As soon as cholera was established in Hamburgh, it appeared evident to us who advocate its contagious nature, that it was likely to be brought in trading vessels to the ports of England which have the most intercourse with that city; and what has been the fact? In those very ports, *viz* Sunderland, Hull and London, the arrival of cholera has been officially announced!—while not a single case has occurred in any of the numerous villages and small fishing towns on the coast of England between Sunderland and Hull, or between Hull and London. And why have all these towns and villages, which on the hypothesis of the diffusion of cholera by the spread of some peculiar atmospheric influence, must have suffered quite as early from this influence as any of the three cities actually affected, why, I ask, have they escaped? The answer is obvious,—because they have no direct communication with Hamburgh.

A melancholy instance of the evil and fatal effects which inevitably follow from an obstinate adherence to the doctrine of the non-contagiousness of cholera, is at this very time exhibited in a convict ship moored in the Thames. A prisoner is attacked with cholera; what means are taken to prevent it affecting his associates? Why they are furnished each with a certain daily allowance of tobacco, and it is soon after announced in all the papers that the smoking has proved quite a luxury to them, has the best effects on their spirits, and has effectively neutralised the fluvatile malaria. The triumph has been but short-lived, and King James himself could not have set forth a more effectual conterblast against tobacco than that which issues from the spirit of the following paragraph:-

Woolwich, October 13, 1848.

The cases on board the convict ship Justitia, up to this day, are twenty-five, six new cases having been reported during the previous twenty-four hours; of that number five have died, and one has been discharged; the other eighteen are not apparently in any immediate danger, but are so debilitated that their medical attendants have not considered themselves justified in entering them on the list of recoveries. Standard, October 14th.

Of course Government Commissioners will consider this spreading of the disease in a crowded hulk as a decisive proof of its non-contagiousness! as they have already done with regard to a ship which arrived at Hull. From their report on the latter case, it appears that sailor after sailor died of Asiatic cholera during the voyage from Hamburgh, because, forsooth, they indulged in eating plums and drinking cider. Such indulgences were not likely among convicts on board the hulk, who used nothing unwholesome until they were set smoking by authority!

It is some satisfaction to find Oxenstiern's parvula Sapientia presides over the sanitary affairs of Great Britain; for as soon as it was ascertained that the cholera had safely arrived in London, via Hamburgh, the authorities immediately interfered, and quarantine was established between the two cities!

In conclusion I beg to repeat, that the unanimity of all Government officials called on to report on the non-contagiousness of cholera, is a striking proof that nothing is impossible to English Capital.

I remain, dear sir, faithfully your's,

Robert J. Graves."

These are the outpourings of a thoroughly embitterd man who had separated from his wife, resigned his hospital appointment and become anxious, persecuted and depressed. He was in his early fifties and it takes little imagination to deduce that he was almost certainly suffering from endogenous depression.

Chapter 15

A Sea Change

In recent years, psychiatrists have persuaded us to use the term affective disorders for those three great changes in mood; depression, anxiety and mania. Of these, depression is far and away the commonest, indeed it is estimated by one authority that some forty percent of the population may suffer from it at some time in their adult life. When the condition is full blown it is easily recognised, but in its milder forms it is frequently missed and many a sufferer has been treated for years for a multitude of minor ailments from which such patients often complain. When an attack of depression is severe, the behaviour of the individual is diagnostic and the appearance so tell-tale as to be easily identified, even in a portrait. The word 'attack' is used here advisedly since it is a condition which is capable of reversal, either spontaneously or following treatment. But, and this is a very important proviso, anyone who has had even only a single episode of depression is much more likely to have another attack than one who has not. Some believe that the condition tends to run in families, but this is far from being certain.

When we last visited the Robertsons in Huntingdon Castle, Clonegal, we were able to photograph a daguerrotype of Graves which hung on the staircase. It must be one of the earliest portraits to be made using Daguerre's technique, in Ireland, because it was only in the 1830s that the first ones appeared in Paris where Daguerre was developing his technique with the help of Nièpce. It was a wonderful method for obtaining a true portrait of the sitter and would probably still be in use if it had not been overtaken by the much more convenient method of photography. Like many of the daguerrotypes that have survived from that period, it had been charmingly hand coloured. There sits Graves, slumped in his chair, looking thoroughly miserable and depressed, there is a slight pink flush over his cheek bones, which may or may not be artistic licence, I think not. His features are a little coarse and his eyebrows are virtually absent. It is difficult to believe at first glance that this is the same sitter as the dashing young Graves depicted in Grey's portrait in the Royal Hibernian Academy which must have been sketched in 1822 or perhaps a little earlier.

The findings of coarsening of the features with loss of hair and perhaps the flush over the cheekbones are the hallmarks, when associated with a slow pulse and great tiredness, of failing thyroid gland function, a condition which might well have helped to usher in the depressive illness. This Sherlock Holmes approach to the

portraiture of Graves is certainly reinforced by an even later
portrait which as an engraving shows him looking particularly
gloomy and rather grim, with a heavy square cast to his face.

Marriages bring happiness and sorrow

Whatever happened to Graves there can be no doubt that something
quite dramatic occurred around 1841 when he was forty-five years
old and just about at the peak of his career. First of all consider his
home life and how far it may have contributed to his abrupt
withdrawal from the academic scene. He originally returned from
his great postgraduate trek around Europe in 1820 or 1821 and
having obtained his first hospital appointment at the Meath, he
proceeded to have a whirlwind courtship and married Matilda
Jane. It must have been a marvellously stablising effect in his life

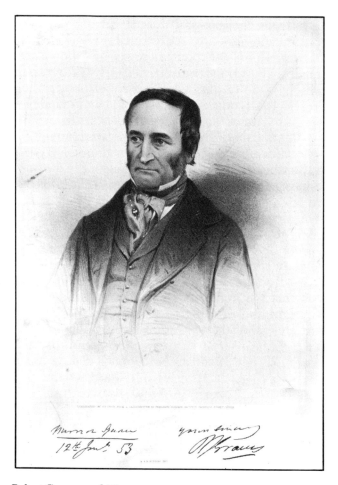

Robert Graves aged 57.

to have, at last, a home and a wife and it seems to have been a happy ménage. Meanwhile he was working something like a twelve hour day and trying to build up a practice and a name for himself in Dublin. He had already started lecturing regularly and within three years we find him helping to found a new medical school in Park Street. Medical schools in those days were not like the ones we recognise today, they merely devoted their energies to instruction in anatomy and physiology and a very little pathology and left the student to attach himself to a hospital or group of hospitals where he could find bedside teaching in clinical medicine. Graves was well known for his grasp of human anatomy and for developmental and comparative anatomy. He also was a life time student of physiology so he was the ideal choice for teaching in such an establishment, but it must also be remembered he still had to cope with his private patients and the rounds in the hospital. Matilda Jane cannot have seen much of her husband and when he did retire to bed it would have been an exhausted head which was laid on the pillow. It was a great thrill when a baby daughter was born after just four years of married life and then the double tragedy, both mother and daughter died. Graves, a deeply religious man, must have found this double blow very hard to sustain.

However he had his work to keep him sane and to prevent him brooding too much on what he had lost; he was in enormous demand as a physician in the city and to cap all this he had started giving his daily lectures at Sir Patrick Dun's which, although time consuming, he clearly delighted in preparing. But even greater comfort came to him in the companionship of Sarah Jane, the daughter of his old friend the Astronomer Royal, Professor John Brinkley, the mathematician at Trinity. Within a year he had married Sarah Jane and once more Graves had a happy home to which to return at the end of each day's work. It is easy to imagine the joy when Sarah Jane became pregnant and what fun they must have had in deciding that if the baby was a daughter then she should be christened Sarah-Jane with a hyphen. It is heartbreaking to contemplate the tragedy when both mother and later daughter died and Graves did indeed have a broken heart. Work for him now became almost his life line and he applied for and was elected to the first full time chair of medicine in Ireland, giving up much of his private practice to do so. The title of King's Professor in the Institutes of Medicine gave him a foot in both the Royal College of Physicians and also the University department at Trinity. He was by this appointment firmly established in the field of academic medicine and it would be difficult to conceive of anyone more suitable for such a position.

To his great delight he found it possible once more to visit the great medical centres of Europe and see some of his old foreign correspondents, friends and teachers, since in the summer vacations

he was able to absent himself from Trinity and his clinical respon-
sibilities were no longer so demanding. So we find him visiting Paris
and Berlin and on at least one occasion going south of the Alps.
Imagine then what a surprise it was when the young professor, he
was only thirty-four years old, announced that he was going to
marry for a third time. We shall probably never know how he came
to wed such a socially conscious young woman as Anna Grogan, the
very smartly turned out daughter of the hunting vicar of Slaney
Park in County Wicklow. She was to bear him six children and
outlive him by twenty years, but what an unusual choice it was for
she quite unashamedly had no use for academic affairs and was a
dedicated social climber, what is more she seems usually to have got
her own way.

Clearly to begin with the marriage was a success, with a family
appearing and then their move to a splendid house in Merrion
Square. Graves seems to have managed to augment his income,
almost entirely by seeing private patients, despite all his other
commitments, and the ascent of the social ladder was all that Anna
could wish for. The stream of distinguished visitors to their house
reaching a proper climax when the Lord Lieutenant and his Lady
sat down to dinner at the Graves' table. At some stage however
there was a break up in the husband–wife relationship and Graves
consoled himself with another woman. For how long this went on
there is no written evidence, but if the story is true, then wife and
husband were eventually reconciled, possibly when Graves first
had signs of the disease which was eventually to kill him. It is clear
that after the fifth child was born there was a twelve year gap before
the sixth, Little Flo, appeared.

Anna was such an unusual partner for somebody like Graves.
She had no compassion and little love, even her children in later
years did not express any affection for their mother, but she was a
wonderful organiser with plenty of style and very good taste. It was
not a warm and caring atmosphere that he could come home to at
the end of a gruelling day's work but rather one where he had to sit
and listen to his wife recounting the day's successes and then
demanding what she expected of him in the coming week. There is
no doubt that social gatherings were of the greatest importance to
Anna and her last twenty years, lording it, if in solitary splendour,
over Cloghan Castle and the surrounding estate down in the west
country were just what she had looked forward to. Her sons left
home early, the elder to enter the church and the second, the army,
while all four girls were married from the castle.

Graves devotes more time to administration
At first irritated and later disillusioned, Graves had eventually left
his wife's side for more congenial and sympathetic company. He was

no longer the enthusiastic and ebullient explorer of all new ideas in science and he was becoming depressed. At the age of forty-five he resigned his chair of medicine which left him more time for other medical pursuits, but then in 1843 he resigned from his beloved Meath Hospital. This really was the writing on the wall and even the pressing requests of his old colleagues could not persuade him to stay. He was devoting more time to the administrative side of the profession and many of his calls were to Kildare Street and the Royal College of Physicians. It was in 1843 also that his colleagues on the council of the College elected him President and this honour he could not refuse, especially as it only involved one year in office. For the next five years after the presidency, he went on working but his papers to the journals were more and more involved in the spread of infectious diseases and trying to persuade his colleagues how cholera and typhus spread, for he was far ahead of his fellows in his understanding of the problems through the experience he had obtained over the years since his first introduction to the subject by Hufeland in Berlin. He had acquired an international reputation and was well known for his work in London. The President of the Royal Society was a friend and in 1849 his name was proposed for Fellowship of that august body which is the ultimate accolade of the English speaking scientific world. In the records of the Royal Society the entry reads as follows:

Robert James Graves Esq,
Merrion Square,
Dublin.
Physician, MRIA. The discoverer of some important points connected with the formation of acid in the human stomach, both in health and disease, and also on some bearings on the functions of the lymphatic and nervous systems. The author of a work on Clinical Medicine, and many essays and detached papers. Distinguished for his acquaintance with the science of Medicine. Eminent as a Physiologist and as a Physician.

Humphrey Lloyd, PRIA. Thomas Andrews. Robert Kane. WF Chambers. RB Todd. W Sharpey. John T Graves. — Richard Bright. Richard Owen. JO M'William. Erasmus Wilson. Golding Bird.

The significance of the names after the —sign is that they were appended by the individuals who attended the Society's House. They are particularly interesting; Bright of Bright's disease was the kidney physician at Guy's Hospital. Richard Owen was the Curator of the Hunterian Museum at the Royal College of Surgeons and later director of the Natural History Museum. Erasmus Wilson was the surgeon anatomist who had Cleopatra's needle brought to London and was President of the Royal College of Surgeons. Graves knew many of them and enjoyed the stimulus of their company and conversation.

Illness looms

Graves was by this time fifty-three years old and although today we would consider him a young man, at that time he would have been treated as very senior, indeed the expectation of life was many years less than it is today. Both of Graves' parents had lived to a great age and so had many of his near relations. However within two years he was suffering from a tumour in the abdomen and spent much time in bed. It was generally considered by his colleagues that he had cancer of the liver which in those days was an unusual diagnosis. Any kind of operation on the abdomen was fraught with danger and was never even contemplated except in the last resort. Certainly no one suggested it on this occasion and my surmise is that as the tumour grew so did the accumulation of fluid within the abdomen. This would have led to great swelling of the ankles and then the legs. Furthermore breathing would have become more and more difficult, even with the patient sitting bolt upright in bed. It was we know from his friends, a painful and distressing way to die, but he remained lucid to the end and welcomed visits from his family and old friends. At the end he asked for celebration of holy communion at the bedside, led some of the prayers himself and finally died quite peacefully.

Anna sold the house in Merrion Square and retired permanently to the country where life at Cloghan Castle was very much her way of life. As a young girl she had been brought up in a country house and she had plenty to do with the family to look after and a very young daughter to bring up. Long and appreciative obituary notices appeared in the national newspapers both in Dublin and overseas because Graves had been a truly international figure in the medical world and the recipient of a number of honorary foreign degrees. In January 1854 the *Medical Times and Gazette* in London published a five page 'Discourse on the life and works of the late Robert James Graves' which had been given by William Stokes who was now Regius Professor of Physic in Dublin. Its delivery had been on the occasion of the meeting of the Association of the King and Queen's College of Physicians in Ireland and it ranged over his whole life, his contributions to medicine and his final illness.

Graves' life comprised three distinct periods

We can follow Graves through three distinct periods in his comparatively short life of fifty-seven years; first we have the brilliant young scientific doctor, well travelled, well informed, with a flair for acquiring foreign languages and with great powers of rhetoric. His only fault seems to have been a trenchant sarcasm and the fact that he simply could not suffer fools gladly.

In his second period he was an outstanding Professor of Medicine who reformed the teaching of medicine to a pattern which has largely stayed unchanged to the present day. He was a world authority on infectious fevers and the manner in which they spread and all this before bacteria and other micro-organisms had even been discovered. His régime of feeding patients who were suffering from fever and preventing dehydration was revolutionary and has saved more lives than anything else he did. He did describe some three patients afflicted with overactivity of the thyroid gland and thanks to Trousseau we still refer to it as Graves' disease although he was not the first to describe it nor particularly interested in it.

Finally the third period of his life was ushered in by depression and was unproductive of new ideas but he was able to play a rôle in management of the health service of Ireland and towards the end of his life he was reconciled with his wife only to succumb to liver cancer at the relatively early age of fifty-seven.

Chapter 16

Graves' Disease

Ask any medical practitioner in Britain, Ireland or the USA what he means by Graves' disease and he will immediately reply that it is the eponym for hyperthyroidism, exophthalmic goitre, thyrotoxicosis or any of the multitude of descriptive names by which this strange condition is known. It is a relatively common complaint in Europe and the USA. With modern methods of diagnosis, such as radioimmunoassay of the level of thyroid hormones in the blood, it may be reckoned to occur as often as one per thousand of the population, if the milder examples of the condition are included.

Whenever a disease earns for itself a host of different names you can be sure that the cause is unknown, and so it is with Graves' disease. That is why eponyms are so useful to the physician because they are usually derived from the name of the first author to describe the condition and thus offer no hint as to the cause. The pattern of signs and symptoms which occurs in such a condition is often referred to collectively as a syndrome, but it will probably come as no surprise to discover that Graves was not the first doctor to describe this syndrome although it is by the application of his name to this one that he is remembered by most people.

Why Graves' disease?
How did all this come about? The blame can be laid fairly and squarely on the broad shoulders of Armand Trousseau (1801–1867) who was both mentally and physically a big man. He came from a medical family in Tours and eventually succeeded to the Chair of Medicine in that prestigious hospital, the Hôtel-Dieu in Paris. He was a contemporary of Graves, an admirer of the Dublin School of Medicine and especially of Graves and Stokes whom he visited and to whose work and writings he always made generous acknowledgement. Trousseau was the first man to open the trachea for relief of obstruction to the airway in diphtheria and his name is still applied to a simple test of compression of the forearm to reproduce spasm of the fingers in tetany. His major contribution to medical literature was his two volume *Clinique Medicale de L'Hotel Dieu de Paris,* published in that city by Ballière in 1862. Another member of the Ballière family settled in London and his successors, carrying the name of Ballière are still publishing medical books in London today. Chapter 72 in the second volume is entitled 'Du Goître Exophthalmique, ou Maladie de Graves' and is written very much in the style of Graves himself, referring as he did, to actual patients in the

wards. Those medical students and doctors who attended the hospital would have seen them earlier in the day as they followed the great man on his teaching round . . . he opens with such a succinct description of the condition and then gives his reasons for calling it Graves' disease, that here are his words quoted in full:

"À numéro 34 de la salle Saint-Bernard, vous avez remarqué une jeune femme dont le physionomie a quelque chose d'étrange. Sa figure offre une expression sauvage, ses yeux sont saillants, son teint est pâle. Elle se plain de battements de coeur; le pouls radial est fréquent, régulier, et présente l'ampleur et la résistance normales. La respiration paraît gênée, et vous avez pu constater une hypertrophie considérable de la glande thyroide. La réunion de ces trois phénomènes morbides: battements de coeur, hypertrophie du corps thyroide et saillie des globes oculaires, constitue une entité morbide dont vous trouverez de nombreuses observations dans les annales de la science et qui a été designée sous les noms de goître exophthalmique, de cachexie exophthalmique, exophthalmos cachectique, de maladie de Basedow etc. . . .

Déjà dans mes leçons cliniques, au mois de novembre 1860, j'ai rappelé en m'appuyent sur le témoignage de Stokes, qu'une grande part de priorité dans la connaisance de cette maladie revenait de droit à Graves (de Dublin). Ceux d'entre vous qui voudrant etre convaínçus à ce sujet, n'auront quà relire *Les Leçons de Médicine Pratique* de Graves, et le chapitre du goître exophthalmique dans l'ouvrage de Stokes sur les maladies du coeur."

But Trousseau's fellow countrymen in France did not follow his lead nor did the medical profession in any other European country. It is only in those primarily English speaking areas of the world that physicians followed Trousseau in using the eponym of Graves' disease.

Parry first described the syndrome
The credit for the first to describe hyperthyroidism is more properly accorded to Caleb Hillier Parry who was born in Gloucestershire and studied medicine at Edinburgh. He went to school with Edward Jenner the pioneer of vaccination and they remained friends for life, indeed Jenner dedicated his most famous work, *Inquiry into the Causes and Effects of Variolae Vaccinae*, which established vaccination as the means of preventing smallpox infection, to "CH Parry MD at Bath, My Dear Friend". Parry settled in Bath, then a fashionable spa, and established a huge and indeed lucrative practice being brought into relationship with many of the most prominent citizens of the day, at a time when it was fashionable to be seen taking the waters in the pump room. It is recounted that once, while walking home with a companion after a long morning's work, his friend remarked that his waistcoat pockets, cut large

according to the fashion of the day, seemed quite full, possibly of guineas. "Yes," replied Parry. "I believe there are ninety-nine; I may make it a round sum before I get home".

But Parry, in addition to being a successful doctor was also a careful clinical observer and researcher making major contributions to medical knowledge. He was one of the first to draw attention to the narrowing of the coronary arteries in angina pectoris and described other pathological conditions of the heart valves. Some of his most important papers were published posthumously by his son in 1825 and it is in them that we find a description of a group of patients with what we should really refer to as Parry's disease but in practice today call Graves' disease. His account starts thus: "There is one malady which I have in five cases seen coincident with what appears to be enlargement of the heart, and which, so far as I know, has not been noticed in that connection by medical writers. This malady to which I allude is enlargement of the thyroid gland". He described eight cases in all, one with severe exophthalmos, the condition in which the contents of the orbit are thrust forward so that the patient has a permanent stare.

All this information giving the correct priority to Parry was fully available some eighty years ago in Sir William Osler's great textbook of medicine, which was the standard work for very many years in all English speaking countries. No heed was taken of it and Graves' disease remains as the most commonly used descriptive term to this day.

Graves' description of the syndrome

Graves' description of the malady, which was from then on to bear his name, first appeared in the *London Medical and Surgical Journal* in May 1835. The article is entitled 'Newly observed affection of the thyroid gland in females' and has the sub-heading: 'From the clinical lectures delivered by Robert J Graves, MD, at the Meath Hospital, during the session of 1834–1835. Because it was this publication which became the reason for Graves' name being attached to the disease, although by no means his most important contribution to medicine, the opening paragraph of the article is reproduced here:

"I have lately seen three cases of violent and long continued palpitations in females, in each of which the same peculiarity presented itself, *viz* enlargement of the thyroid gland, the size of this gland, at all times considerably greater than natural, was subject to remarkable variations in every one of these patients. When the palpitations were violent the gland used notably to swell and become distended, having all the appearance of being increased in size in consequence of an interstitial and sudden effusion of fluid into its substance. The swelling immediately began to subside as the violence of the paroxysm of palpitation decreased, and during the intervals the size of the gland remained stationary. Its increase of size and the variations to which it was liable had attracted forcibly the attention both of the patient and their friends. There was not the slightest evidence of anything like inflammation of the gland."

He goes on to say . . . "may be considered as indicating that the thyroid is slightly analagous in structure to the tissue properly called erectile".

Basedow credited in Europe

It would be churlish at this juncture not to mention Basedow, for it is his name which today is applied to the condition in most other European countries. Carl A von Basedow was the son of an aristocratic family and was born in 1799 at Dessau and subsequently studied medicine at the university of Halle. His special interest was surgery and he spent two years in what today we would call postgraduate study in the surgical service of two famous old Paris hospitals; the Charité and the Hôtel Dieu. Returning to his native Germany in 1822 he settled in Merseburg, practising as Kreisphysicus or district physician, an appointment which included the duties of general physician, general practitioner and surgeon. It is often forgotten in these days of the National Health Service in Britain with its accent on specialisation, that formerly much of the surgery which was performed away from the major cities was carried out by general practitioners. Many of these men, for there were no women surgeons in the nineteenth century, did their operations in cottage hospitals or the patient's own home, and it was only with the advent of the NHS in 1948 that they had to choose a career exclusively in either surgery or general practice.

Basedow, as well as becoming a much loved and respected figure who was devoted to the welfare of his fellow citizens of Merseburg had clearly been imbued in his university days with the investigative spirit. Unlike most physicians at that time, he performed his own post-mortem examinations and was able to describe his findings in the papers which he wrote on a number of different diseases. His prime contribution in the thyroid field appeared in 1840 entitled *Exophthalmos durch Hypertrophie del Zellgewebes in der Augenhohle* which may be translated as exophthalmos due to hypertrophy of the cellular tissue in the orbit. In this he propounded what was to become known as the Merseburg Triad of exophthalmos, struma and palpitation of the heart; struma is the old Latin-derived word for thyroid enlargement or goitre.

Basedow's interest in toxic goitre was unflagging and in 1848 he published the autopsy findings on a patient who died from exophthalmic cachexia or in other words gross hyperthyroidism which if untreated makes the patient look as wasted as the inmate of a concentration camp.

Sadly it was his interest in the post-mortem findings or morbid anatomy as the subject is usually called that was his undoing. In 1850 he pricked his finger in the post-mortem room when examining a patient who had died of typhus and he succumbed to septicaemia at the early age of fifty-five.

Graves' many gifts to medicine

It really is rather unfortunate that Graves' name should have been perpetuated in the medical profession by applying it to a condition which he was certainly not the first to describe nor indeed one in which he showed particular interest. I have found no other references to it in his published works. But although Graves' great admirer Trousseau said that exophthalmic goitre should be known as Graves' disease, it is true, as Wolstenholme points out, that Graves was the first to describe angio-neurotic oedema thirty years before Quincke, to whom we usually give the credit. For good measure he also clearly recorded intermittent pallor of the fingers and toes some twenty years before Raynaud, although this is always referred to now as Raynaud's phenomenon. He was among the first to point out the value of fresh air, good ventilation and a full diet in the treatment of pulmonary tuberculosis or pthisis due to which some seventy thousand people a year were then dying in the British Isles; but above all 'he fed fevers'. On the other hand we can be grateful that in dubbing hyperthyroidism Graves' disease, it has at least drawn attention to one who in so many other ways is deserving of our interest. It was Graves, *primus inter pares,* who inaugurated those golden years of Irish medicine in the nineteenth century and this is in no way to belittle the outstanding contributions of his contemporaries, Cheyne, Stokes, Adams, Corrigan, Colles and many others who have left their mark on medicine, often eponymously.

Graves' unique gift to his profession was his superb teaching of clinical medicine at the bedside by which he was not only able to convey to his pupils his own mastery of observation, interpretation and diagnosis, but at the same time to demonstrate how this could be achieved while maintaining high ethical standards, kindness and compassion. Despite the histrionic talents which he undoubtedly possessed, he always managed to be both very observant and critical and with his strongly held Christian beliefs and innate goodness, inspired not only the patient, but those around him with faith and hope. There are numerous examples of students whom he had taught remaining devoted to him for the rest of their lives, passing on his precepts to the next generation of doctors; as for example William Osler so generously admitted. Ireland, with her small population has always been a great exporter of doctors who have ended up practising their skills in every corner of the globe. They took with them to the bedside Graves' tradition of skill, science and compassion which was to have far reaching consequences in hospitals and medical schools all over the world.

Sir William Osler, the Canadian born physician who was Foundation Professor of Medicine at Johns Hopkins University in Baltimore and then Regius Professor of Medicine at Oxford from 1905–1919 spoke of the imperishable glory associated with the names of Robert Graves and William Stokes whose works today are "full of lessons for those of us who realise that the best life of the teacher is in supervising the personal daily contact of patient with student in the wards." He was speaking at the bicentenary celebrations of the medical school at Trinity College, Dublin in 1911 and he closed with a very personal touch: "This is a graduates' dinner, and at last I come to a part of the toast which I know at first hand. Graduates from this School have been much in my life. To usher me into this breathing world one of them came many weary miles through the backwoods of Canada. Across his tie, as he called it, John King MA, TCD birched into me small Latin and less Greek. I owe my start in the profession to James Bovell, a kinsman and devoted pupil of Graves, while my teacher in Montreal, Palmer Howard, lived, moved and had his being in his old masters, Graves and Stokes".

The story of how Osler did indeed owe his start in medicine and much else besides to Dr Bovell and then to Palmer Howard at McGill and so directly to Graves was retold by Harvey Cushing in the opening chapters of his compelling biography: *The Life of Sir William Osler.*

Graves' disease and its treatment

What then is Graves' disease? Briefly, we do not know but we do know how it affects the patient and that is an oversecretion by the thyroid gland, that structure shaped like the letter H which lies in the front of the neck just below the Adam's apple. The thyroid is one of the family of endocrine glands which produce internal secretions or hormones, the word internal referring to the fact that their products pass directly into the blood stream. In the case of the thyroid there are two principal hormones: thyroxine called T4 for short because it contains four atoms of iodine in each molecule; and tri-iodothyronine or T3, with three atoms of iodine. The effect of T4 and T3 is to speed up the metabolic processes throughout the body. A good analogy is the control of ventilation in a solid fuel stove. When the ventilator is opened, more oxygen enters and the fire burns more brightly giving out more heat. The thyroid hormones have just such an effect on every cell in the body. Thus when there is an increase in the secretion from the thyroid, the heart beats faster and more strongly, the individual feels hot, sweats and is apprehensive, the bowels are open more frequently and much urine is passed so that there is constant thirst. As a result the appetite is voracious and the patient is always hungry, hates hot weather, cannot sit still and the hands, moist with sweat, often shake. The eyes appear bright and have a starey look; occasionally, but fortunately rather rarely, the whole contents of the orbit swell and the eye is thrust forward giving the person the most striking appearance. Graves' disease is much more often seen in women than men and tends quite often to occur in more than one member of the same family. The normal thyroid is itself under the control of another hormone which is secreted by the pituitary, a small gland looking somewhat like a cherry on a stalk on the under surface of the brain. This in turn is under regulation by a part of the brain itself so that the endocrine system is in part controlled by the central nervous system. In Graves' disease all this control is lost.

The treatment of Graves' disease is principally by drugs which reduce the manufacture of thyroxine and tri-iodothyronine in the thyroid and it is remarkable how effective one or two tablets taken every eight hours can be. An improvement is noticed in days, and in weeks the patient feels perfectly normal. The tablets are usually continued for about two years and then discontinued; those with mild Graves' disease may have permanent relief, but the more severe ones relapse and are then treated either by a surgical operation to remove a large part of the gland or alternatively, since the late 1940s, by radioactive iodine. It is remarkable how successful all these three methods are in making the patient well and often a combination of more than one kind of treatment serves best. There is one particular complication which is common to all forms of treatment and that is that with the passage of time the thyroid function may fall to limits which are insufficient for the body's needs and so the patient slows up, appears older than their reported age and may even appear prematurely senile. It only requires the taking of thyroxine by mouth to remedy the situation, but occasionally the condition goes unrecognised.

Chapter 17

What is Graves' Disease?

A Little Science

At this juncture it appears only right to ask the questions: what is Graves disease? and what is its cause? Certainly there has never been any lack of researchers working on the problem be they clinicians, laboratory workers or both, since that original description by Graves in the *London Medical and Surgical Journal* for 1835. Indeed in the last forty years there has been a veritable explosion of laboratory investigation in the field as new techniques and research tools have become available.

Endocrinology, which provides one of the fastest growing edges of today's medical research, has been the proving ground for at least three of the new techniques which have revolutionised thinking amongst doctors since the war. First the use of paper chromatography for the separation of the amino acids was immediately exploited by thyroidologists to trace the formation of the thyroid hormones, as internal secretions from the endocrine glands are called, and led to the discovery in 1951 at the National Institute for Medical Research at Mill Hill in London by Rosalind Pitt-Rivers and Jack Gross of the most active member, tri-iodothyronine or T3. The arrival of radio-active isotopes to label chemical processes in the living body was at first largely a tool for thyroid workers since radio-active iodine was easy to produce in the atomic reactor and its commonest isotope, ^{131}I, had a convenient half-life for the researcher of eight days. For the first time, with the assistance of autoradiography, the investigator could actually produce a pictorial record of what iodine was doing in the thyroid since wherever the isotope was incorporated in the gland it blackened the photographic film placed in contact with it. From there it was only a short step to mapping the thyroid's activity in the neck and then to treating Graves' disease with larger and therefore more energy-bearing doses. The credit for being the first to do this goes to the late Dr Saul Hertz of Boston whose brother's name is better known from his car hiring firm.

The first demonstration of auto-immunity

Probably the biggest contribution that the thyroid was to make in pioneering new technology was in the field of immunology. This old established subject was reborn in the war years when Peter Medawar demonstrated how skin grafts from donors other than the host were rejected, the only exception being grafts from one identical twin to another, because identical twins have identical immunological systems. This was eventually to lead to the first successful kidney transplant between identical twins and then to the long haul in matching the donor's kidney to the recipient patient and latterly suppressing the immunological processes which reject it.

The surprising break through which followed was the clear demonstration in man that some individuals actually overstep nature's immunological defences and begin rejecting their own tissues. This so-called auto-immune process was first demonstrated in the thyroid in 1956 by Ivan Roitt and Deborah Doniach in patients with failing thyroid function due to Hashimoto's disease. Hashimoto was a Japanese surgeon who reported in 1912 the thyroid changes in a common affliction typically seen in women in their forties in which there is insidious destruction of thyroid function with a slowing down of all the bodily processes from mental to physical. It also occasionally occurs in men and rarely in children.

These immunological changes, both protective and destructive are largely mediated by globulins secreted by highly specialised white blood cells. The immunoglobulins, or Igs for short, are complex molecules and according to their actions they are designated by the capital letters of the alphabet, IgA, IgB, IgC and so on. The ones primarily involved in thyroid disease are IgGs (immunoglobulin G) but they are many and various and one of the more exciting discoveries was that some of them can stimulate the thyroid abnormally. But how? That is the burning question.

Onset and course of Graves' disease

Now to the first half of the query with which this chapter started, which was: what is Graves' disease? Well, it is the condition of hyperthyroidism, characterised by an increased secretion rate of thyroid hormones with a sustained raised level in the circulating blood. Certain families carry a genetic trait which makes them more susceptible to it and although it is more frequently diagnosed in those countries where medical and especially diagnostic services are well developed, it does appear to occur more often in those individuals of European descent wherever they may be living.

The onset of Graves' disease can be quite rapid in the young, over a period of a few days or weeks, but in older patients whose tissues are no longer so responsive, the onset can be insidious and thus make diagnosis more difficult. The level of thyroxine or T4 and the more potent tri-iodothyronine or T3 is elevated in the circulating blood and there is evidence that T4 can be broken down or transformed into T3 in the tissues where these hormones work; the amount of T4 and T3 can be readily estimated in today's laboratory from a small blood sample. The increase in the hormones as they circulate in the blood in turn stimulates the metabolic process of every cell in the body. The pulse quickens in rate, the increase in nervous energy makes the patient over anxious, the fingers tremble and may even lose their grip on the teacup. Unnecessary heat is generated and the body tries to cool itself by producing sweat and the kidneys produce more urine leading to frequency in passing it and thus thirst develops. The superabundant energy means that on a normal diet there is loss of weight and the muscles seem to lose their power so that climbing the stairs is very wearying. The bowels work overtime and some patients with Graves' disease first consult their doctor because of severe and persistent diarrhoea.

One of the most striking features of the whole condition is the shining of the eyes which become more prominent as they are thrust forward by increased muscle tone and the increased bulk of the tissues in the bony orbit. In a tiny group of patients this prominence of the eyeball progresses out of all proportion to the other signs of the disease and may be so gross that the eyes' survival is even jeopardised; the paralysis of eye muscles in such individuals is an added and crippling disability. Some researchers, in particular Brown Dobyns in the USA, proposed a separate hormone which affects the eyes, but although an assay was devised for this, the theory remains unconfirmed and the present view of endocrine exophthalmos suggests an autoantibody antigenic to material in the orbit as a cause.

Proposed explanations

What theories have been proposed in the last 150 years to explain all these unusual phenomena? At first it was thought that the pituitary hormone which controls the thyroid, the so called thyroid stimulating hormone or TSH, was being produced in excess; but when assay techniques became available the converse was discovered. Then in 1956 two workers in New Zealand, Adams and Purves, discovered that if some serum was taken from a patient with Graves' disease and injected into a mouse it caused prolonged stimulation of the animal's thyroid, this being in contrast to the brief stimulation which normal human TSH produced. The new substance was named LATS or long acting thyroid stimulator and subsequent work in the laboratory revealed that it was an immunoglobulin of the IgG variety which latched on to the thyroid in the same way as an antibody, but how it combines with the thyroid cell membrane is still not clear. As it is an immunoglobulin, LATS is now referred to as a Thyroid Stimulating Immunoglobulin or TSI, in other words an autoantibody. Studies on patients with Graves' disease showed that only about fifty percent of them had this TSI in their blood, but this is not so surprising since antibody and antigen are reacting from such different species as mice and men. Further studies on those patients with Graves' disease who did not have

TSIs showed that they did have a substance circulating in their blood which inhibited the binding of TSH to their thyroid tissue and the new substance was at first called LATS-protector and this proved to be yet another IgG.

The problem thus appeared to be related primarily to the receptor sites in the thyroid where these abnormal stimulators latch on in competition with the body's own normal stimulator i.e. TSH. The concept of the Thyroid Receptor cells having specific Antibodies, TRABs, thus arose.

It is now known that lymphocytes fall into two main groups: T-lymphocytes (or thymus lymphocytes) and B-lymphocytes (or bursa lymphocytes). It would be the T-lymphocytes which were at fault and clones of abnormal T-lymphocytes have been found in some families which would explain the genetic pattern of Graves' disease and the observation that in such patients the thymus is often enlarged and of an abnormal pattern under the microscope. It was the great Australian immunologist Sir Macfarlane Burnet who pointed out that the thymus is like the finger print of the individual in the way that it controls the destiny of circulating lymphocytes or white cells, especially this particular group which are called T-lymphocytes.

The classification of human beings into various categories according to their immunological response, by studying the reaction of their white cells to a wide spectrum of antibodies has resulted in what is known as the HLA system. At first it seemed that those with the HLA B8 group were much more at risk to develop Graves' disease, and those who were additionally DW3 were most susceptible, but real interpretation and significance of this work is yet to be clarified.

Enough however has been said to show that the disease to which Parry, Graves and Basedow first drew doctors' attention is a fascinating disarrangement of the body's immunological system and one whose cause is still unsolved. How fortunate that it masquerades under a variety of eponymous names which serve splendidly as a disguise for our ignorance. It is just possible that the immunological changes which have been discovered may only accompany or reflect the causes of the disease rather than be the cause itself.

In the 1960s I proposed the idea that Graves' disease was a highly conditioned form of neoplasia. The reasons for this were that I had been interested in the 1890–1910 reports in the literature of the treatment of patients with Graves' disease by feeding them with raw thymus (sweetbread—or more correctly heartbread). I repeated some of this work and also studied the histological changes in samples of thymus removed from patients whom I operated upon for Graves' disease. I wrote to Sir Macfarlane Burnet at that time who replied "I find it very interesting. I can never resist trying to twist any such ideas to my own point of view". He continued, "so here are a few remarks which may or may not be relevant: I like to think of 'true' malignancies as starting from a single cell and extending from it—here one would almost have to assume an initiating hormonal (?) stimulus which pushed all or nearly all the cells into, shall we say 'neoplastoid' (sic) activity in which they are unresponsive to the normal controls. In the highly active toxic thyroid I can easily conceive that a surface antigen specific to the thyroid cell which is virtually never released in the normal gland is released to the draining lymph nodes and initiates both thymus-dependent and thymus-independent responses. The first would provide the cells that initiate the lymphocytic infiltration and the second, LATS." Sir Macfarlane Burnet was not only an FRS, but joint winner of the Nobel Prize with Sir Peter Medawar for his work in immunology. Even so, such a theory does require a lot of imagination.

Finally, Graves' disease is occasionally accompanied by soft tissue changes in the body especially exophthalmos or protrusion of the eye-balls, pre-tibial myxoedema which is overgrowth of the tissues over the shins and ankles, and acropachy or thickening of the tissues of the fingers. TSIs have been shown to bind not only to the thyroid but also to certain other tissues such as fat cells. This is auto-immunity at its most self-destructive level. Clearly an enormous amount of research is needed to elucidate the mechanisms involved and then at last it may be possible to devise rational methods of dealing with the root cause of these disabling, if rare, complications.

Envoi

An Appraisal

Any account of Graves and his contributions to medicine must face up to the problem of what happened to him in his middle forties which completely altered the pattern of his life style. From then on he made less and less contribution to medical science, became cantankerous, highly critical of those around him, and finally withdrew prematurely from the professional positions he had long held in the university and hospital. This was also the time when he broke with his wife. In addition to all this, contemporary portraits show a surprising alteration in his physical appearance.

It is tempting to draw an analogy with Richard Bright the equally brilliant physician at Guy's Hospital in London who apparently similarly neglected his large and very attractive family but persisted in going to great lengths to care for his patients. This is not so rare an occurrence among consultants whom I have known and I really do not know why they behave in this way unless it be a great urge to acquire fame, or far less likely, wealth. Milton certainly acknowledged its existence:

"Fame is the spur which the clear spirit does raise,
(That last infirmity of noble minds)
To scorn delights and live laborious days."

As a young man, Graves was immensely outgoing; all his colleagues and friends commented on his superabundant energy and confidence in what he did, even his writings at that time reflect this. Clearly he was verging on the condition that psychiatrists would call hypomania and such a mood is indeed one that may eventually dip into depression. The more manic that individuals are, the more likely they are to become so severely depressed that they finally commit suicide. Certainly Graves did not fall into that category but something brought about a great change of character as he approached fifty years of age. That is an age when sexual drive in many men begins to lessen and it has even been dubbed the male menopause, although I find this a poor analogy. There was, in Graves' case, a very clear change of character, a sea change, and contemporary portraits give good evidence of failing thyroid function in the coarsening of the features and evidence of obesity. What a tragic fate for one whose name was ever after to be linked to overactivity of the thyroid.

No doubt the character of his wife Anna must, as time went by, have been an accessory factor in driving him into depression. She was incapable of love in the warm protective way he craved and her social climbing and denigration of scholarship eventually estranged him altogether. Anna, tiny, good-looking, with a tough hard character, no interest in intellectual affairs but with admirable taste in artistic matters was not the right wife for him.

Richard Bright of Guy's, who took the trouble to go and vote for Graves to be made a Fellow of the Royal Society was so like him in many ways. Brilliant in everything he touched, as a young man he travelled widely like Graves; one time accompanying Sir George Mackenzie on a scientific expedition to Iceland. He likewise married young and having fathered a large family would always plead pressure of medical duties and then neglect his wife and children. Bright's great great niece, who trained as a nurse and as an author, has recently written the biography of her distinguished ancestor and is at a loss to explain his distant attitude to his own family when his kindness and consideration for his patients was such a feature of his public life. Like Graves he was a very private person and was equally aloof, he also had his personal papers destroyed. I consider both doctors represent a pattern of behaviour which is not so unusual as it is claimed to be.

Brilliant student and natural philosopher

The young Dr Graves was a striking personality, tall, dark haired, with flashing eyes and a very animated way of expressing himself. He had always been top of his class at school, a gold medallist at Trinity and equally brilliant as classicist and in medical school. To these rich gifts must be added that of eloquence to which the Irish brogue adds a certain golden timbre, and his daily lectures at Sir Patrick Dun's Hospital were the talk of the town, and this in Dublin in the 1820s was praise indeed. He was of a serious turn of mind and apart from his great affection for his brother Hercules, seems usually to have preferred the company of older men. He was never a ladies' man nor a frequenter of the drawing rooms of Dublin, which in his day were like courts for anyone who was socially conscious.

His three years of postgraduate study in Europe, a true hegira in those days of difficult travel, moulded his character and influenced the rest of his professional life more than anything else he ever did. Indeed he continued for the rest of his years to correspond with distinguished colleagues overseas and occasionally he made further visits to Europe to talk with them. It may well be that in studying Graves for so long, I too have become imbued with the analogic method and see similarities perhaps rather too often, perhaps indeed where they do not exist, but Graves' early life was moulded by his travels just as Charles Darwin's was by his voyage in the 'Beagle'. There are certainly other interesting parallels between the lives of these two scientific thinkers who contributed so much to the advancement of knowledge in the nineteenth century.

At heart Graves was a true natural philosopher in a period when that subject was just beginning to blossom. In addition he not only loved to use his classical knowledge but was equally at home when looking at biological problems; geology, chemistry, or epidemiology—he was a natural enquirer. However, like a true physician, when confronted with a patient he became totally involved in the individual and thus his contributions to the medical literature were not only very practical in terms of treatment, but show that he never lost the common touch. He became involved in every detail of prescribing and nursing and, in addition, the psychology of dealing with the relatives. When an epidemic of typhus struck the undernourished population in the west of Ireland he immediately volunteered in a practical way and went to Galway with a team of assistants. He was fearless in this regard and that at a time when many doctors were dying from the contagion.

Outstanding Career

His return to Dublin in 1821 from his travels must have caused quite a stir in the rather closely knit profession of the day. Here was a brilliant and talented young man with good connections and better informed about new advances in medicine in Europe than anyone else. His gift of eloquence and powerful presence swept most people off their feet and he was almost at once elected to the staff of one of the city's most prestigious hospitals which had only just been rebuilt, the Meath. There and at Sir Patrick Dun's Hospital he practised for the rest of his professional life. Within two years he had been elected a Fellow of the College of Physicians and a year later he was co-founder with his colleagues of a new medical school in Park Street. Simultaneously he was elected as a lecturer in the Institutes of Medicine. On top of all this he proceeded to found the new *Dublin Journal of Medical Science* and remained as its co-editor for very many years. With his burgeoning private practice, and many patients will always flock to a new doctor because he is new, he at once was a force to reckon with in both town and gown. With his excellent and very practical papers appearing in the medical journals every few months and his lectures each evening at Sir Patrick Dun's, he was the leading spirit in those Golden Years of Irish Medicine which positively scintillated with men of talent whose names are still household words the world over from their eponymous links with disease: Stokes, Adams, Corrigan, Cheyne, Colles, to mention only the most famous. Graves, Stokes and Colles are still often referred to as the great Triad of Irish Medicine.

He had not been back a year in his home city when he married Matilda Jane Eustace, but within four years she was dead along with their daughter Eliza. Within a year he again plunged into matrimony with Sarah Jane who was the daughter of John Brinkley the Professor of Astronomy, an outstanding mathematician who had come to Dublin from Cambridge. A stimulating intellectual he became a friend of Graves, with whom he cooperated in the field of probability in relation to epidemic diseases. But tragedy struck again and Sara Jane died within the year as did her baby daughter. At this time Graves clearly immersed himself in his work but once again he essayed matrimony, and his choice of Anna, the daughter of the Revd Grogan of Slaney Park, very much the county family, seems perhaps out of character. However, they had six children, two sons and four daughters, and she outlived him for twenty years.

There were of course flaws in Graves' character and the greater the man the greater the attention and condemnation that such weaknesses are likely to receive. He did not suffer fools gladly and when he was critical he sometimes spoke out far too clearly with his strictures, whilst his sarcasm could be searing. But to his credit he never bore a grudge and even his slanging match with Corrigan in the columns of the *Dublin Quarterly Journal of Medical Science* contains generous admission of the latter's great contributions to the organisation of improved health services in the Irish community. In his youth and as a young consultant he was probably too quick to draw analogies where sometimes they did not really exist, but this approach to natural phenomena was often one of his strengths as it certainly proved to be later in the hands of Charles Darwin. His essays, whether on the problems posed by the salinity of the Dead Sea on its flora and fauna, or the progress of Asiatic cholera across the Western World, show the impact of an original mind.

His greatest gift to the medicine of his day was his revitalisation of the system of clinical or bedside teaching which was a subject long neglected. The manner and quality of his teaching was greatly enhanced by his continuing involvement in research allied with a warm compassion for his patients, attributes which are as necessary today as they were then. The clarity of his written word produced the standard text on clinical medicine to be used for many years, not only in the British Isles and North America, but through translations in France, Germany and Italy. He pioneered studies on the spread of infectious diseases both in his own country and on a broader canvas, worldwide. Above all he was the epitome of a good physician.

The final illness
There is only one account extant of his final illness and death, it is

in the conclusion of Stokes' biographical preface to the volume entitled *Graves' Studies in Physiology and Medicine*. Stokes was his pupil, colleague and devoted friend, and it is appropriate that their statues still stand side by side in the hall of the Royal College of Physicians of Ireland in Kildare Street in Dublin. Here is his account:

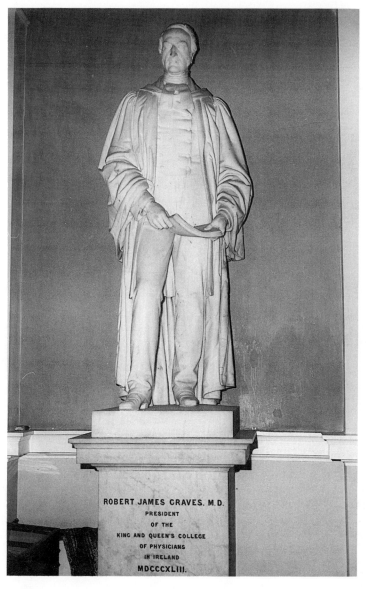

ROBERT JAMES GRAVES, M.D.
PRESIDENT
OF THE
KING AND QUEEN'S COLLEGE
OF PHYSICIANS
IN IRELAND
MDCCCXLIII.

The posthumous statue of Graves by the Irish sculptor Joy, which stands in the Hall of the Royal College of Physicians of Ireland.

"It was in the autumn of 1852, he being then in his 57th year, that the symptoms of the malady, which was to prove fatal, first showed themselves. In the following February he began to succumb to the

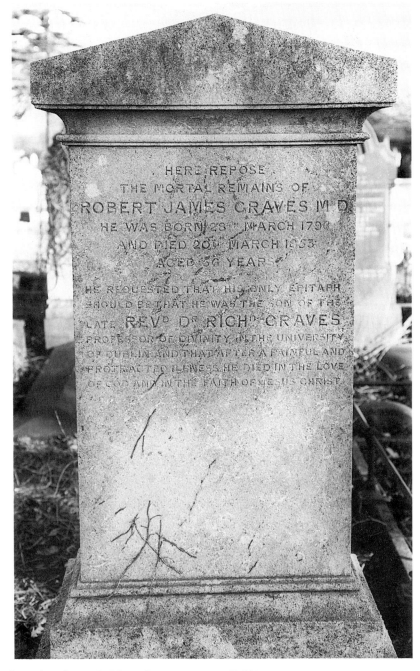

Graves' tombstone in Mount Jerome cemetery, Dublin.

disease. Although at times his sufferings were great, yet he had many intervals of freedom from pain. And he then showed all his old cheerfulness and energy. To the very last he continued to take pleasure in hearing of any advance of knowledge that tended to ameliorate the condition of man, or to throw light on his relations to a future state. In this latter point of view, the discoveries of Layard greatly interested him, as illustrative of the Sacred History; and thus he was permitted to fill up the intervals of his sufferings, even to the last; for his mental faculties never failed or flagged, a mercy for which he often expressed a fervent gratitude; and so he was providentially enabled to review the past, and to form a calm and deliberate judgement on the religious convictions of his earlier years. And once the truthfulness of these was ascertained, he adhered to them with that earnestness which characterised all his decisions. It was after the attainment of this state of patient expectation that one who was dear to him expressed a prayerful wish for his recovery, "do not ask for that," he replied, " it might prove a fatal trial".

"His mind having become thus satisfied he made few remarks on these subjects, except in reply to the enquiries of others. Thus, when referred to the prophetic illustration of purifying and redeeming love, "a fountain shall be opened for sin and for uncleanness," "No," he said, "not a fountain, but an ocean".

"On the day before his death he desired (a second time) to partake of Holy Communion with his family. When some explanations were commenced he answered, "I know all that; I do not regard this as a charm, but I wish to die under the banner of Christ". Feeling himself sinking, he asked for a prayer, and a petition was offered suitable to his condition; but he seemed to long for something more, and when questioned, replied, "I want some prayers that I know, some prayers of my youth, some of my father's prayers". The Litany was commenced, he immediately took up the well known words, and when the speaker's voice faltered, he continued them alone, and distinctly, to the end of the strain, "Whom thou hast redeemed with thy most precious blood".

"On the 20th day of March 1853, and without renewed suffering, he ceased to breathe.

"His tomb is in the cemetery of Mount Jerome in Dublin. It bears the following inscription, dictated by himself:

Robert James Graves
Son of Richard Graves, Professor of Divinity
who
after a protracted and painful disease
died in the love of God, and
in the
faith of Jesus Christ.

References

The major sources of information are given here under chapter headings.

Chapter 1
Introduction

Means JH. A Sentimental Journey. *The News.* Massachusetts General Hospital, Boston, Jan 1961.

Means JH. *The Thyroid and its Diseases.* (2nd ed.) Philadelphia: Lippincott, 1948.

Holograph letter from Dr Howard Means, Sept 15 1963.

29 Montgomery Street, Bangor, Maine.

Dear Selwyn,

I want your advice on a literary project—its worthwhileness. I find that I thoroughly enjoy writing and I want to do more of it. Actually it has occurred to me that it would be a fitting climax to a career in thyroidology to write a brief biography of Robert Graves. He strikes me as having been a great figure in medicine quite apart from exophthalmic goiter.

It would be great fun for me to do this if it hasn't been done already, and I have not discovered that it has, and if this is correct I would love to undertake it. Among other things it would provide a good excuse for me to spend some time in Dublin and perhaps Edinburgh (where he went to medical school) and London. All of this would be pleasant. Do give me your candid opinion about whether all this makes sense to you. I am aware that you know much about Ireland and Irish medicine and I shall greatly value your opinion.

If it is favourable to the project I shall probably be after you later to direct me toward source material. There is good precedent for going into medical history in one's latter years, namely Popsey Welch who became very busy with medical history in his last decade.

My kindest regards to Ruth and yourself.

Ever yours,
Howard Means.

Graves R J. *Clinical Lectures on the Practice of Medicine.* (2nd ed.) Neligan JM, ed. 2 vols. London: The New Sydenham Society, 1884.

Graves RJ. *London Medical and Surgical Journal* 1835;7: 516.

Parry CH. *Collections from the unpublished papers of the late Caleb Hillier Parry.* vol 2. 11–128. London: Underwood, 1825.

Flajani G Obs. LXVII. In, Collezione d'osservazione Reflessioni di Chirurgia. *St Michele A Ripa Plesso Lino Con.* Vol 3. 270. Roma. 1802.

Basedow von CA. Exophthalmos durch hypertrophie des Zellgebes Augenhohle. *Wochenschr Ges Heilkunde,* 1840; **13**: 197–223.

Chapter 2
Graves' Forbears

MacDonnell, Hercules Henry Graves. *Some Notes on the Graves Family*. (For Private Circulation Only). Dublin: Browne and Nolan Printers, Nassau Street, 1889.

Holograph Stemmata of Nora Kathleen Parsons whom on Oct 15 1912 intermarried with Manning Durdin Robertson. Manuscript book held by the Robertsons of Huntingdon Castle, Clonegal, Co Carlow.

Robertson, Nora. *Crowned Harp. Memories of the Last Years of the Crown in Ireland*. Dublin: Allen Figgis, 1960.

Hammond EP. St Lawrence's Church: Mickleton (including Hidcote Bartrim) Gloucestershire. (2nd ed.) Stratford upon Avon: George Boyden Ltd, Rother Street, 1980.

Hammond EP. *Mickleton and its Church Memorials and Hatchments*.

Personal communication from Doctors Donald and Jennifer Olliff. *The Story of Our Village*. Mickleton Womens Institute, Glos. recounts how in 1885 the façade of Mickleton Manor was transported on a railway to nearby Kiftsgate House.

Chapter 3

Growing Up

Wilson TG. (President of the Royal College of Surgeons in Ireland 1958–60). *Victorian Doctor. Life of Sir William Wilde*. London: Methuen, 1942.

Dictionary of National Biography. Life of the Very Rev Richard Graves. London: Smith & Elder.

Graves RH. *Richard Graves DD. Dean of Ardagh and Regius Professor of Divinity in the University of Dublin*. (Collected works with a memoir of his life and writings by his son.) 4 vols. Dublin. 1860.

Chapter 4

Trinity College Dublin. Europe in Turmoil

Kirkpatrick TPC. *History of the Medical Teaching in Trinity College Dublin and of the School of Physic in Ireland*. Dublin: Hanna & Neale, 1912.

Maxwell C. *A History of Trinity College Dublin (1591–1892)*. Dublin. 1946.

Pyle F. *Trinity College Dublin*. Dublin: Eason & Son, 1983.

Newman JH. *The Idea of a University*. London: Longman Green, 1907.

Newman Charles. *The Evolution of Medicine in the 19th Century*. p95. Oxford University Press.

Wilde WRW. *Biographical Memoir of the late Robert J Graves*. Dublin: McGlashan & Gill, 1864.

Stokes W, ed. *Studies in Physiology and Medicine by the late Robert J Graves.* London: John Churchill, 1863.

Churchill WS. *A History of the English Speaking Peoples.* Vol 3. p 239. London: Cassell & Co, 1957.

Stubbs JW. *The History of the University of Dublin.* Dublin: Hodges Figgis, 1889.

Dungannon Convention and Grattan's Parliament. Facsimile documents published by the National Library of Ireland.

Chapter 5
Medical School

O'Brien E. *Conscience and Conflict: A Biography of Sir Dominic Corrigan 1802–1880.* Dublin: Glendale Press, 1983.

Cameron CA. *History of the Royal College of Surgeons in Ireland and of the Irish Schools of Medicine.* Dublin: Fannin & Co, 1886.

Fallon M. *Abraham Colles 1773–1843.* London: William Heinemann Medical Books Ltd, 1972

Fleetwood J. *History of Medicine in Ireland.* Dublin: Browne & Nolan, 1951.

O'Brien E, Crookshank A, Wolstenholme GW. *A Portrait of Irish Medicine.* Dublin: Ward River Press, 1984.

Chapter 6
Graves in Europe
The Men Who Shaped His Career

Blizard Sir William. In: *Plarr's Lives of the Fellows of the Royal College of Surgeons of England.* d'Arcy Power, ed. London. 1930.

Professor Stromeyer. In: Hirsch A. *Biographisces Lexicon.* Berlin: Urban & Schwarzenberg, 1929–1934.

Professor Johann Blumenbach. Trans, Bendyshe T. *The Anthropological Treatises of Johann Blumenbach.* London: Longmans, 1865.

Freedman BJ. Caucasian. *British Medical Journal* 1984; **288:** 696–698.

Professor Christoph W Hufeland. In: *Dictionnaire de la Médècine chez Bechet Jeune.* Paris. 1828.

Professor Behrend. In: *Dictionnaire des Sciences Médicales.* Paris: CLF Panckouke, 1832.

Professor Johannes Colsmann. In: Dahl-Iversen E, ed. *Festkrift udgivet af Kopenhavns Universitet.* Copenhagen. 1960.

Chapter 7
Traveller's Tales
Graves Making the Grand Tour

Stokes W. Biographical Notice. ppIX–LXXXVIII. In: *Studies in Physiology and Medicine by the Late Robert James Graves.* London: John Churchill & Sons, 1863.

Armstrong Sir W. *Turner.* London. 1902.

Powell Cecilia. *Turner in the South.* London.

Reid Sir George. JMW Turner. In: *Encyclopaedia Britannica.* London. 1947.

Wilde WRW. *Biographical Memoir of the late Robert J Graves.* Dublin: McGlashan & Gill, 1864.

Chapter 8
The Traveller Returns
The Meath Hospital

Widdess JDH. *The Meath Hospital and County Dublin Infirmary 1753–1900.*

Ormsby Lambert. *History of the Meath Hospital.* (2nd ed.) Dublin. 1892.

Boxwell William. Historical Sketch of the Meath Hospital. *Medical Press & Circular* **207:** 206–24.

Graves RJ. *Clinical Lectures on the Practice of Medicine.* 1 chap 1. Dublin. 1848.

Forbes J. *A Treatise on Diseases of the Chest.* (In which they are described according to their anatomical characters and their diagnosis established on a new principle by means of acoustic instruments.) London: T & G Underwood, 1821.

Laennec RTH. *Traité de L'Auscultation Medicale.* Paris. 1819.

Osler W. Speech at bicentenary of the Medical School of Trinity College July 6th 1912. Quoted in: Cushing Henry. *The Life of William Osler.* London: Oxford University Press. 1924.

Chapter 9
Graves as a Family Man

Professor Brinkley. In: *Dictionary of National Biography.*

Welcome to Cloghan Castle. Lusmagh, Banagher, Co. Offaly: 1973. Published for visitors to the castle.

Soully, James. *The History of Cloghan Castle.* Banagher, Co. Offaly.

The Landed Gentry. Facsimile documents published by the National Library of Ireland.

Robertson, Nora. *Crowned Harp. Memories of the Last Years of the Crown in Ireland.* Dublin: Allen Figgis, 1960. Particulars of the Parsons family.

Meenan FOC. The Georgian Squares of Dublin and their Doctors. *Irish Journal of Medical Science* 1966. **484:** 149–54.

Chapter 10
Graves as His Contemporaries Saw Him

Fallon M, *The Sketches of Erinensis.* London: Skilton & Shaw, 1979.

Widdess JDH. *The Royal College of Surgeons in Ireland and its Medical School.* (2nd ed.) Edinburgh: Livingstone, 1967.

Radbill SX, ed. The Autobiographical Ana of Robley Dunglison. *Transactions of the American Philosophical Society* 1963: **53** pt8: 120.

Graves states in the first edition of his *Clinical Medicine* that his publications in: *Dublin Hospital Reports, Dublin Medical Journal* and *London Medical Gazette* were often translated into French, German and Italian and had also been collected in a book published in Philadelphia by Doctor Robley Dunglison.

Our Portrait Gallery, No 27, Robert James Graves MD. *Dublin University Magazine* Feb 1842; 260–73.

Wilde WRW. *Biographical Memoir of the Late Robert J Graves MD.* Dublin: McGlashan & Gill, 1864.

Duncan JF. The Life and Labours of Robert James Graves. *Dublin Journal of Medical Science* 1878; **73:** 1–12.

Stokes W. A Discourse on the Life and Works of the Late Robert James Graves. *Medical Times and Gazette* 1854; **184:** 1–5.

The Statue of Doctor Graves. A leader in: *British Medical Journal* 1877; **22:** 12.

Chapter 11
The Four O'Clock Lectures and Sir Patrick Dun's Hospital

Moorehead TG. *A Short History of Sir Patrick Dun's Hospital.* Dublin: Hodges, Figgis & Co, 1942.

Brent P. *Charles Darwin. A Man of Enlarged Curiosity.* London: William Heinemann, 1981.

Darwin Charles. *The Voyage of the "Beagle".* London: Amalgamated Press, 1905.

Kirkpatrick TPC. *History of the Medical Teaching in Trinity College Dublin.* Dublin: Hanna & Neale, 1912.

Stokes W, ed. *Studies in Physiology and Medicine by the Late Robert J Graves.* London: John Churchill, 1863.

A Portrait of Irish Medicine. O'Brien E, Crookshank A, Wolstenholme GW, eds. Dublin: Ward River Press, 1984.

Chapter 12
Graves as Author
See Graves' Bibliography p151

Chapter 13
Clinical Medicine
Graves' Magnum Opus
Clinical Lectures on the Practice of Medicine by Robert J Graves first appeared in Dublin in 1843. The second edition which increased to two volumes was revised by J Moore Neligan and Graves dedicated it to the Rt Hon William, Earl of Rosse, President of the Royal Society, when it was published in 1848.

The work was translated into French and published with a glowing foreword by Graves' admirer A Trousseau in Paris. Translations into both German and Italian are reported but I have not seen copies of them.

The commonest edition which is available today is the reprint by The New Sydenham Society in London in 1884 which is in two volumes and bears an English translation taken from the *Medical Times and Gazette* of Trousseau's introduction to the French edition.

Chapter 14
1846 Famine and the Corrigan Affair

Edwards RD, Williams FD. *The Great Famine. Studies in Irish History* 1845. Dublin. 1956.

Woodham-Smith Cecil. *The Great Hunger Ireland 1845–9.* London: Hamish Hamilton, 1962.

History of Irish Pestilences. Reports on the Tables of Deaths. l part v; 191. *Census for 1851.*

O'Brien E. *Conscience and Conflict. Biography of Sir Dominic Corrigan.* Dublin: Glendale Press, 1983.

Report of Board of Health and College of Physicians Dublin quotes Graves' argument with Corrigan.

Lambard HC. Open letters to Dr Graves. *Dublin Journal of Medical Science* (a) **10:** 17–24. (b) **10:** 101–105. 1836.

Chapter 15

A Sea Change

Shakespeare's *Tempest*
Full fathom five thy father lies;
of his bones are coral made.
Those are pearls that were his eyes:
Nothing of him that doth fade,
But doth suffer a sea-change
Into something rich and strange.

Widdess JDH. *Annals of the Meath Hospital and County Dublin Infirmary 1753–1900.*

Annals of the Meath Hospital—Meath Hospital Annual Report for 1951. Dublin 1952.

Collis M H. *A lecture given at the Meath Hospital 1867.* Dublin. 1867.

The Minute Books of the Meath Hospital contain the correspondence with Robert Graves when he resigned from the staff.

Chapter 16

Graves Disease

Graves RJ. *London Medical and Surgical Journal.* **7:** 516.

Trousseau A. *Clinique Médicale de L'Hôtel-Dieu.* 2 tomes. Paris: Baillière, 1862.

Parry CH. Collections from the unpublished work of the late Caleb Hillier Parry. **2:** 11–128, London: Underwood, 1825.

Basedow von CH. Exophthalmos durch hypertrophie des Zellgebes in der Augenhohle. *Wochenschr Ges Heilkunde* 1840; **13:** 197–223.

Cushing H. *William Osler.* London; Oxford University Press, 1924.

Graves' Bibliography

All the works recorded here are ones which I have been able to locate and read, the majority of them being in the library of the Royal College of Surgeons of England in Lincoln's Inn Fields in London. They have an outstanding collection in the history of medicine as well as surgery and the biological sciences. Where I have been unable to handle the actual book or paper, that fact is recorded.

I realise that such a list is practically never complete and I would welcome information from anyone who can draw my attention to omissions and how I can amend them.

Graves RJ. Report of the fever lately prevalent in Galway and the West of Ireland. *Transactions of the King and Queen's College of Physicians in Ireland* 1824; **4:** 408–36.

Graves RJ. On the effects produced by posture on the frequency and character of the pulse. *Dublin Hospital Reports* 1830; **5:** 561–71.

Quotations from Graves and Stokes. Diseases of respiratory organs. Diseases of the abdominal viscera. *London Medical and Surgical Journal* 1830, **5:** 457–68 and **6:** 1–12.

Graves RJ. Observations on secretion and the intimate structure of glands. *Dublin Journal of Medical Science* 1832; 1: 42-56.

Graves RJ. Observations on the treatment of various diseases. *Dublin Journal of Medical and Chemical Science* 1832; 1: 144-56.

Graves RJ. Observations on the treatment of various diseases, continued. *Dublin Journal of Medical and Chemical Science* 1832; **1:** 286–304.

Graves RJ. On double and single vision. *Dublin Journal of Medical and Chemical Science* 1832; **1:** 255–65.

Graves RJ. Observations on the treatment of various diseases. *Dublin Journal of Medical and Chemical Science* 1833; **2:** 14–27.

Graves RJ. Observation on the treatment of various diseases. *Dublin Journal of Medical and Chemical Science* 1833; **8:** 151–73.

Graves RJ. Observations on the treatment of various diseases. *Dublin Journal of Medical and Chemical Science* 1833; **2:** 167–80.

Graves RJ. Observations on the treatment of various diseases. *Dublin Journal of Medical and Chemical Science* 1833; **3:** 353–70.

Graves RJ. Chronic purpura cured by corrosive sublimate. *Lancet* 1832–1833; p268.

Graves RJ. Observations on the treatment of various diseases. *Dublin Journal of Medical and Chemical Science* 1834; **4:** 309–28.

Graves RJ. *A Lecture on the Functions of the Lymphatic System.* (2nd ed.) Dublin: Hodges & Smith, 1834.

Graves RJ. Newly observed affection of the thyroid gland in females. From the clinical lectures delivered by Robert J Graves MD at the Meath Hospital during the session 1834–35. *London Medical and Surgical Journal* 7: 1835; 516–17.

Graves RJ. Clinical Lectures at Sir Patrick Dun's Hospital. *London Medical and Surgical Journal (Renshaw)* 1834–35; 7: 801-7.

Graves RJ. Observations on the treatment of various diseases. *Dublin Journal of Medical and Chemical Science* 1835; 6: 49–74.

Graves RJ. Notices concerning works on the practice of physic, surgery, pathology and physiology recently published in Germany. *Dublin Journal of Medical and Chemical Science* 1836; 8: 116–35.

Graves RJ. On tympanitis occurring in fever, and the different modes of treating it. *Dublin Journal of Medical and Chemical Science* 1836; 8: 499–504.

Graves RJ. On a peculiar affection of the nerves of the teeth. *Dublin Journal of Medical and Chemical Science* 1836; 9: 1–5.

Graves RJ. On the use of tartar emetic combined with opium in certain varieties of delirium occurring at an advanced stage of continued fever. *Dublin Journal of Medical Science* 1836; 9: 211–38.

Graves RJ. Cases of violent delirium, occurring at an advanced stage of maculated or typhous fever and treated successfully by doses of tartar emetic frequently repeated. *Dublin Journal of Medical Science* 1836; 9: 449–66.

Graves RJ. Observations on the treatment of various diseases. *Dublin Journal of Medical Science* 1837; 11: 391–408.

Graves RJ. On the state of the pupil in typhus and the use of Belladonna in certain cases of fever. *Dublin Journal of Medical Science* 1838; 13: 351–66.

Graves RJ, Stokes W. Dr Clutterbuck versus the stethoscope. Dr Hope on auscultation in valvular disease. *Dublin Journal of Medical Science* 1839; 14: 178–80.

Graves RJ. Observations on the treatment of various diseases. *Dublin Journal of Medical Science* 1839; 14: 349–93.

Graves RJ. Sketch of the origin and progress of Asiatic cholera. *Dublin Journal of Medical Science* 1840; 16: 355–432.

Graves RJ. Appendix to report on the progress of Asiatic cholera. *Dublin Journal of Medical Science* 1840; 17: 98–105.

Graves RJ. Observations on the treatment of various diseases. *Dublin Journal of Medical Science* 1840; 18: 225–60.

Graves RJ. Case of very long continued epilepsy without any appreciable lesion of the brain or spinal marrow. *Dublin Journal of Medical Science* 1840; 17: 372.

Graves RJ. Sketch of the original progress of Asiatic cholera. In; Ashwell Samuel *et al. Medical and Surgical Monographs.* Philadelphia: Waldie, 1840.

Graves RJ. On purpura haemorrhagica and a newly observed species, Exanthema haemorrhagicum. *Dublin Journal of Medical Science* 1841; 18: 260–77.

Graves RJ. On the treatment of various diseases. *Dublin Journal of Medical Science* 1842; **20:** 385–422.

Graves RJ. On the treatment of certain affections of the heart. *Dublin Journal of Medical Science* 1842; **21:** 181–206.

Graves RJ. *Clinical Lectures on the Practice of Medicine.* (1st ed.) Dublin: Fannin & Co 1843. (In America 3 editions of this work appeared between 1843 and 1848.)

Graves RJ. On pericarditis. *Dublin Journal of Medical Science* 1843; **23:** 162–3.

Graves RJ. On the races of mankind. *Dublin Literary Journal.* April 1844.

Graves RJ. On the law which regulates the relapse periods of ague. *Dublin Quarterly Journal of Medical Science* 1846; **1:** 59–76.

Graves RJ. Observations on the nature and treatment of various diseases. *Dublin Quarterly Journal of Medical Science* 1847; **3:** 324–47.

Graves RJ. A letter to the Editor of the Dublin Quarterly Journal of Medical Science relative to the Proceedings of the Central Board of Health of Ireland, with postscript. *Dublin Quarterly Journal of Medical Science* 1847; **4:** 513–44.

Graves RJ. Fever and its spread in the 1847 epidemic. *Dublin Quarterly Journal of Medical Science,* 1848; **5:** 30.

Graves RJ. On the contagion of Asiatic cholera. *Dublin Quarterly Journal of Medical Science* 1848; **6:** 289–316.

Graves RJ. Letters on cholera. *Dublin Quarterly Journal of Medical Science* 1848; **6:** 475–6.

Graves RJ. *Clinical Lectures on the Practice of Medicine.* (2nd ed.) (2 vols.) Dublin: JM Neligan, Fannin & Co, 1848. (This is the definitive review of the work with an update on the treatment of cholera and fever as practised by Graves in the *Dublin Quarterly Journal of Medical Science* 1848; **7:** 421–7.

Graves RJ. On the progress of Asiatic cholera. *Dublin Quarterly Journal of Medical Science* 1849; **7:** 1–39.

Graves RJ. Observations on cholera, especially on its mode of propagation. *Dublin Quarterly Journal of Medical Science* 1850; **10:** 257–86.

Graves RJ. Observations on the nature and treatment of various diseases. *Dublin Quarterly Journal of Medical Science* 1851; **11:** 1–20.

Graves RJ. Postscript to Doctor Graves' paper on cholera. *Dublin Quarterly Journal of Medical Science* 1851; **11:** 214–17.

Graves RJ. On the nature and treatment of epilepsy. *Dublin Quarterly Journal of Medical Science* 1852; **14:** 257–64.

Graves RJ. On the application of Gutta Percha in the treatment of diseases of the skin. *Dublin Quarterly Journal of Medical Science* 1852; **14:** 1-9.

Index